PERFECT
BALANCE

DAVID MOORE

ISBN 978-1-63844-297-4 (paperback)
ISBN 978-1-63844-298-1 (digital)

Christian Faith Publishing, Inc.
832 Park Avenue
Meadville, PA 16335
www.christianfaithpublishing.com

Printed in the United States of America

This book is dedicated to my father, Walter Milner Moore, who taught me about balance, weighing all options and then deciding that if the best option were not present, create one. He lived his life seeking to achieve balance in everything. He was probably a workaholic when young but slowed the pace in aging and retired to enjoy over thirty years in the golden age. He was my hero in reminding me that life is choices and seeking the balance will help you make the right choice. It gave me faith, hope, and a strong work ethic.

CONTENTS

Foreword..9
Preface..11
Introduction..13
Resolutions..17

Chapter 1: Balance: You Learned Everything You Need to
            Know in the Third Grade....................................19
    Happiness 20
    Willpower 20
    Salvation 20
    The Difference 21
    Lifelong Journey...21
    Truth..23

Chapter 2: Eat Right...24
    Water 27
    God Cures..29
    Smoothies 30
    Inflammation 30
    New Ideas 31
    Big Family..31
    Love Life 32
    Proper Nutrition 33
    Artificial Sweeteners (Sugar Substitutes) 33
    Restaurants..35
    Water Types...35
    Pregnancy..36
    Detox 36
    Choices 38

Hygiene..39
Pam's Story..39
Fasting...40
Prioritize 41
Variety...42
Eating by Blood Type 42
Fried..43
Sugar 44
Vision 46
Self-Healing 46
Caffeine...47
Bread...48
Obesity 48
Lectins 49
Vegetarian 51
Juicing...52
Minerals 53
Supplements and Vitamins..53
Dental 54
Fruit..54
Moderation 56

Chapter 3: Drugs 58
Male-Enhancing Drugs 59
Diet Pills 60
Environment..61
Technology...63
Television 63
Alcohol and Tobacco 64
Charcoal...65
Cures...65
Sun..66
Parkinson's...67
Genetics 68
Immune System 69
Age..70
Future 70

Chapter 4: Get Enough Sleep 73

Chapter 5: Exercise..79
    Breaking the Chains 80
    Stretching...82
    Weight Training 91
    Cardio..92
    Colonoscopy 93

Chapter 6: Wash Your Hands 94
    Animals...94
    Routine 95
    Time 96
    Addictions...97

Chapter 7: Love God...100
    Joy...103
    Love and Marriage..104
    Equally Yoked 105
    Financial 106
    Destiny or Fate...106
    Research on Willpower...107
    Silence..109
    Open Mind...110
    Choices 110
    Prayer and Chain and Ring 111
    Forgiveness...111
    Beyond Control 113
    Major Truths 113
    Soul...114
    Awareness...115
    Positive Thoughts...118
    Intentional 119
    Attitude..120
    Rationalize 121
    Rules 121
    Pain...123
    Filters 124

Expectations 125
Stress 125
Forgetful 127

Chapter 8: Entertainment 129

Chapter 9: Home Remedies 130
Research on the Body..138
Age..144
Food that Heals..145
Elimination 146
Awareness...147
Perfection 151

Chapter 10: Scriptures and Inspiration.........................155

Personal Note..157
Conclusion..159
Acknowledgments 163

FOREWORD

For most of my life, I have encouraged anyone who would listen to pay attention to what they are doing to the body and for the body, to fuel it properly on the inside and out, to treat the body as a temple of God before waiting for a scary health crisis to occur. I have also encouraged others to be proactive with their learning, their health, understand how to anchor healthy habits, control negative thinking, how to get the body moving daily, how to build deep relationships, and at the same time be a strong witness and follower of Jesus Christ. During my life, I have met a lot of people who talk about healthy living, healthy giving, spiritual abundance, and how to live a joy-filled life; however, none come close to living by the standard of excellence like my friend David Moore.

I met David many years ago. He appeared at first like he had a perfect life and a perfect past. After learning more about his early beginnings, how he navigated uncertainty, hardships, and trials, with the principles of health talked about in his book, and crediting the source of his strength being the Lord, I knew he would write a book someday. David Moore has tremendous insight and passion to help others, not just live an average life but the best life ever imagined.

Many health books on the market are complicated, confusing, and leave out Christ completely. David has found a way to simplify and clarify true principles, save time for the reader by not only extrapolating from the most influential leaders on wellness but providing his own success blueprint on how to make decisions, take personal responsibility for all parts of life, define the true definition of willpower, and lean on the Lord for one's constant companion and complete source of strength. This book contains the nuggets of wisdom from hundreds of health books and religious interpretive books, as well as personal life experiences. It also removes the superfluous material that might hinder you getting a grasp of what's important.

David is a stalwart example of health, spiritual living, and abundant giving. He says, "Believe you can change. Decide to make that change. If you truly love yourself the way God loves you, you will make that change to be a healthier, happier person. The human potential can reach amazing heights, especially when plugged in to God."

I am impressed with the wisdom, dedication, and encouragement contained in this book. I implore you to read this book and implement his suggestions. The payoffs will be well worth the price of sacrifice. When you have health, anything is possible; and without it, nothing else really matters.

Dr. Rachel Smartt ND, smartttransformations.com
Author, speaker, plant-base coach, nutritional counselor
Peachtree City, Georgia

PREFACE

You learned everything you need to know in the third grade. Eat right, get enough sleep, exercise, wash your hands, and love God. Loving God is most important, but in this order, the core (eat right, get enough sleep, exercise) will help you love God in a way that may surprise you.

Congratulations. You have made the first step by selecting this book toward a better life. The purpose of this book is to help the reader save time reading hundreds of books by using the nuggets of wisdom in this book. The advice in this book can save you thousands of dollars being spent on health care.

If you want to be healthier or if you suffer from any illness or disease, keep reading. This book will give you great ideas to accomplish what you need to be healthy *and happy*. Each area of the eating right, getting enough sleep, exercise, staying clean, and loving God can be achieved.

Be an EAGLE!
Eat right.
Always get enough sleep.
Get to exercising.
Love cleanliness.
Especially love God.

INTRODUCTION

I love people. I am one of eleven children. Through this experience, I learned DNA and genetics play an important part in who you are. I also experienced many people who said they are the way they are because of their parents. Those same people, after being tired of being unhealthy, many obese, made a decision to change. They changed their lifestyle, lost weight, started eating a better diet, and therefore were able to sleep better, and exercise. DNA and genetics need not limit you!

Their simple decision to change their lifestyle resulted in them being nothing like their parents. They were healthy, happy, and continued to live many years beyond the age their parents lived. If someone has genes that dictate there should or will be a problem, that is all the more reason to make the right choices to live a healthy life.

God wants to give you wisdom, so you know how to acquire that willpower, to make the right decisions. Don't worry. You will not be asked to buy any supplements or anything else. Most people just change what they were buying from processed food to whole real fruits and vegetables.

Exercise is not hard, and it is not work. If you think so, you are doing too much for your current condition. My workout can be as long as two hours, but I have been exercising all my life with an average of three times per week. You need to have the right attitude to exercise. Know that it will definitely give you peace of mind eventually, eliminate impurities in your body, stimulate digestion, increase your capacity to work, and give you an all-over good feeling. For most of my life, it has also given me a feeling like I am superman. Many of my friends can tell you that I have often replied to their general question about "how are you doing" that I am fabulous, marvelous, fantastic, or that I am superman. I genuinely feel this way every day. Don't hate me. You can feel this way. I genuinely love my fellow man, and that is why this book went to print. Please receive it in the spirit in which it is written.

Your mind communicates with every cell in your body constantly. The neurotransmitters in your brain are the essential molecules that enable your brain to function. They are everywhere in your body. Your attitude and beliefs are determinative to your health. Your immune response is ready, willing, and able to do what it needs to do, but any bad choices you make will hinder its effectiveness. Choices make all the difference in the world.

The science of medicine still has many uncertainties. A cold virus only makes some people sick, but not others. Standard medical treatments are unpredictable in many cases. Some treatments actually make patients worse. Alcohol, tobacco, and most drugs are toxins to your body.

Seven reasons medical care stops working: The doctor doesn't know what caused your illness. No drug or surgery will correct it. Treatments are too risky, toxic, expensive, or all three. Side effects outweigh the benefits. The condition is too far advanced to be reversed. You're too old. The doctor made a mistake.

Although people live longer today, many suffer with bad health and/or disability. Two-thirds of cancers are preventable. An estimated 440,000 people die every year due to medical mistakes in US hospitals alone. Many go unreported. This should get your attention.

My heart goes out to all who have cancer. I know sometimes cancer can occur when you are doing the right things. This is why we can benefit from EAGLE, doing what we can, especially in those two-thirds of the cases.

The total direct expense of adverse events as medical mistakes is known and estimated at hundreds of billions of dollars annually. Indirect expenses such as lost economic productivity from premature death and unnecessary illness exceed $1 trillion per year, *$1 trillion.*

Writing in the journal of the American Medical Association in 2009, Dr. Tait Shanafelt says numerous global studies involving nearly every medical and surgical specialty indicate that approximately one of every three physicians is experiencing burn out at any given time. That number rose to 54 percent in 2014. Many physicians are not mentally alert when treating you.

If you have an illness that has advanced to the point that EAGLE is not helping, I highly recommend *The Healing Self* by Deepak Chopra, MD, and Rudolph Tanzi, PhD, 2018. You will be achieving lifelong wellness following the short time it takes to read this book.

Determination, persistence, fortitude, and a desire to achieve are labels you may consider. Whatever the label is that brings to mind what you need to change in your lifestyle, choose that one. I chose to get mean (determined) in order to prove to my friend, the doctor who challenged me to a detox, to prove to him that I could do it, man-to-man. Whatever incentive you need, use it to get a healthy and happy life.

I may hold some punches but not many. Most people would rather die than change their diet. And most do sooner than they should. Save yourself and the ones you love with the hidden healing powers disclosed in *Perfect Balance*. Find relief from hundreds of symptoms and conditions.

RESOLUTIONS

If you dislike making New Year's resolutions and it is near the first of the year, make this change anyway! I have made great changes in health near the first of the year. They were not resolutions per se, but a change that benefited me, and I did not let any stigma prevent me from claiming that benefit! Never be superstitious. It is a waste of mental thinking.

A conscious effort was made to have the research information in a separate part of the book so you may be fed first only what is needed to make you healthy. Your curiosity about the research can be answered later. You certainly can get anything on the Internet, just be careful. Many sites lead with a great story to finally offer to sell you something, usually a supplement.

Be sure to read the ingredients in supplements. You may find that you are allergic to some of the ingredients. You can make a conscious effort to shift away from the old paradigm of traditional medicine. You should only seek drugs and surgery after you've tried holistic medicine and, first, the plan in this book.

If you identify with other seekers of higher consciousness, you can embrace personal transformation as a major goal in your life and seek to do that as quickly as possible. You can and should view your body as being tied to a spiritual journey. After all, God made you, and you are his temple.

As you clean your diet, you will become transformed, one step at a time. For example, eliminate one food that will make you feel better. This will be sufficient for that time. This should give you vision to continue. Continue eliminating foods that do not agree with your body until you reach optimum health.

Seize the faith you have. That is also the knowledge which you use to continue. Have faith in the process. Have faith in the results you're seeing, even if small. Have faith in yourself. This process can be easy and even fun, if you expect good results.

This book was written for you. I have yet to find someone who could not benefit from these nuggets. One day you will be overjoyed from the health that will exude from your body!

Balance

My father, Walter Moore, an entrepreneur and salesman, taught me more about balance than anyone. He was always espousing Dale Carnegie's book *How to Win Friends and Influence People*. Dad gave me the desire to be a businessman; and my mother, Caroline, led me to the knowledge of God. It was a balance that allowed me to prosper, a perfect balance that enabled me to achieve a happy and healthy life every day. I want you to have the same or a similar balance that is right for you.

I had a strong desire to work hard from a young age and actually started working part-time when I was nine years of age and full-time seven days per week when I was eleven years of age. My father's teaching instilled in me a good work ethic. My mother taught me the spiritual balance. She and others actually dragged us to church when we were young because we did not want to go. However, the preacher was able to pierce that resistance, and I accepted Jesus.

I was transformed forever. Jesus said, "Whoever acknowledges me, I will acknowledge him before the Father [God]." This information is disclosed to you so you understand I believe not only your physical health is very important but also your mental and spiritual health. Knowing and loving God truly and completely can heal you completely.

Happiness

When you clean your diet and get enough sleep and exercise, you will be able to choose your attitude daily.

Willpower

Willpower is the function of blood sugar. Worth repeating: willpower is the function of blood sugar. You get your blood sugar right by doing a detox or some form of changing your body clock. When your blood sugar is right, you can choose to be happy.

This willpower is not only for choosing the right foods, but for everything in life. You can then choose whatever you wish (more about willpower later).

Salvation

The most important thing in your life is salvation. People say it is to glorify God. What better way to glorify God than to accept his son as your savior? People say it is to know God. What better way to know God than to have a personal relationship with Jesus? Life is meaningless without Jesus and your salvation.

There is a scripture in the Bible that says, "Have the attitude of Jesus." Jesus Christ always had an attitude of doing what God the Father wanted. God wants us to be healthy and happy. That is why he sent Jesus. The Bible is the Word of God and is God, which is truth.

There is scripture talking about sacrifice and suffering. If you have the right attitude, you realize that although sacrifice and suffering might be inevitable, you can choose to see those as a gift. The gift from God is giving you wisdom. Look for the good in everything.

The Difference

God, give me the courage to change the things I can, the serenity to accept the things I cannot change, and the wisdom to know the difference. Choose now to live healthy. Good things will follow. Great things will follow.

During my life, I have watched many Christians eat unhealthily and have serious illnesses. I understand that you can have a sickness or illness that is not caused by your diet. In this book, I will be discussing the ones that are caused by your diet.

When I hear people say it was not diet but a virus. Did you ever stop to think that maybe it was the bad diet that lowered the immune system that allowed the virus to take control? Why do so many people get sick and others do not in the exact same circumstances? For example, with a simple cold virus, a healthy person's immune system wins the fight and does not get sick. I tell you the truth, diet is more important than most can imagine.

Miracles are real. They happen daily. However, why take a chance on wanting God to heal something that could've been prevented by your choices to eat healthy?

I apologize for sounding harsh. However, I want you to understand that you have two choices: eat healthy and live healthy or not. Many can claim an exception. Those are usually the same ones not willing to try a good clean diet for several weeks. The ones who do make it happen are usually amazed.

Lifelong Journey

If you have already chosen to eat healthy but still have some problems, choose today to continue the tapering effect to improve even more. This is a lifelong journey. You can choose daily to make the right choices. Make God choices.

Laughing at yourself is a good way to not get stressed. I always say "too blessed to be stressed." My good friend Pastor Dr. Gary Howard taught me that. Actually, you can practice laughing at little things, not just big jokes. The more you laugh and smile, you will be less stressed. Choose to smile even when others may not. The only time I get close to being stressed is when I go to a doctor and too much blood is taken (my opinion)!

Simply anticipating bad events in the future creates a level of stress in the body and mind and can create anxiety or even physical pain. I am not saying that going to the doctor is a bad event, but some people may experience a negative feeling by just thinking about going to a doctor. The term psychosomatic refers to real physical symptoms that arise from or are influenced by the mind and emotions rather than a specific organic cause in the body (such as an injury or infection). Get your mind right by starting with the EAGLE plan.

When completely healthy, you can choose or have the willpower to ignore future bad events. It sounds like a miracle, and in today's society, it is. It will not hurt you to do the EAGLE plan and see if it works for you.

EAGLE
Eat right.
Always get enough sleep.
Get to exercising.
Love cleanliness.
Especially love God.

Some experts believe that people overrate their happiness. You can actually and truly be happy when you are healthy—healthy in body, mind, and soul.

Truth

Who am I? A child of God. God loves you and wants you to be healthy and happy. If you are honest and truthful with everybody, especially yourself, you will feel like Jim Carrey's character Fletcher Reede in the movie *Liar Liar*. He said, "This truth stuff is pretty cool." It is actually life-changing.

There is still much value in the printed book. You may have it with you at all times, not depending upon electricity or batteries. You can mark, highlight, and underline easily or quickly for future reference. This book gives hope. It does this by bringing nuggets of wisdom from one hundred other books.

Eat Right

Diet means the kinds of food that a person habitually eats. Every person has a diet. You learned everything you need to know in the third grade: Eat right, get enough sleep, exercise, wash your hands, and love God. Love God is priority, but if you don't do the others, your time to love God will be shortened. Your quality of life will certainly be less. Eating right is absolutely first to get yourself in a healthy state, physically and mentally. This order is most important because if you do not eat right, you normally will not sleep right; and if you do not sleep right, you don't feel like exercising. It all starts with what goes in your mouth.

If you are eating right and still unable to sleep, do some strenuous exercise even if just before bedtime. When I was young, if this happened, I would do push-ups until I could do no more. I would fall into the bed and fall asleep immediately.

Never feel tired again. Read on. There are so many wonderful books on diet. I will not reiterate what everyone knows. However, you are what you eat. You are also what you eat/ate. Animals ate some diet, and now you eat them. Think about it. Some people eat beef that is organic, which should be better than the other beef. Whatever the animal ate is now in you. That is why so many healthy people never eat pork. I will add to that. Any beef that is not the best, like filet mignon with no fat or gristle, is not good for human consumption. Some of the strongest people in the world, the best athletes and deep thinkers, like scientists, are pescatarians. They only eat fruit, vegetables, and fish. One footnote is that people with certain blood types get weak as vegetarians and especially as vegans (only fruit and vegetables).

There was one time in my journey I felt weak, when omitting beef and turkey. However, I was not consuming enough good fish. Always eat wild-caught fish and not farm raised. Now I feel good as a vegetarian, eating only fruit, vegetables, and fish. My splurge is a small piece of filet mignon. Occasionally, I eat turkey. Both will have zero fat or grizzle.

All red meat (beef, venison, lamb etc.), if eaten, should only be no more than once per week or two and in a small portion the size of your palm. My partner Ken Green says that the limitation is a good moderation. He also agrees that most people don't know what moderation means. Remember that gravy on meat or on anything else is not good for humans.

Animals need to be fed good food, freshwater, and feel secure. This fundamental need is true also for humans, and in this order. Once humans have good nutrition and healthy water, they usually feel secure. This security should lead to the next step, getting enough sleep.

When I was young, especially the teenage years and through my twenties, I would eat what everybody else ate, the American diet. Of course, like everybody else, I was sick periodically. Later I realized it was in direct correlation to what I had eaten. Even before my teenage years, at home every Friday, my mom did the grocery shopping; so when we returned home, she made hotdogs. I wish I could tell you these were of the highest quality, but they were not. Later I realized that ironically, whoever had more than two hot dogs, even the adults, would mysteriously be sick later that evening. I mean sick vomiting, every time.

If you listen to your body and have a desire to be healthy, you can adjust your diet by paying attention to how your body responds to what you eat. Listen to your body after eating certain foods, not before. (Listening to your body before may be just a craving). However, common sense will tell you not to consume alcohol, tobacco, drugs, fried foods, and usually caffeine.

Each time you read "listen to your body," it means listen to your body to eliminate foods, not adhering to cravings. Just because the whole world thinks that it is good to do a particular thing, for example have cereal and toast and a piece of fruit in the morning, with coffee, does not mean that is the right thing for you. When your body does not respond ideally to these, it is letting you know it is not right for you. Once again, listen to your body in every situation. You will be amazed how fast your body heals itself, provided you give it good food.

I chose the tapering effect for adapting my diet to getting older. I established some absolutes. The first for me was caffeine. By removing caffeine from my diet, I eliminated heart palpitations (now thirty-five-plus years ago). The next was eliminating carbonated beverages, which just made me feel better longer. I started removing fried foods, which eventually I was able to eliminate totally. This happened following a detox recommended by my friend who is a doctor (more later on detox).

After I reached forty, I realized ice cream seemed to go immediately to my midsection. It appears that for men, it is above the belt; and for women, it is below the belt as weight gain. My friend Alex Heath says, "A moment on the lips and forever on the hips." It can be true for some foods like ice cream. Before I quit ice cream, I could actually feel the difference after a short period of time, around my waist (above the belt).

This moment on the lips is accurate. The taste is in your mouth for a few seconds; but the effect of the bad food can degrade your health for hours, days, or even years. Some absolutes may be needed, which means not consuming any ever, could be caffeine, fried foods, and processed sugar.

When we were young, we ate many bad foods. We were young, strong, resilient, and survived. As you age, your body loses that ability to compensate for bad food. Many people have lost their gallbladders, perhaps your warning mechanism. I never read ingredients until I was sixty years of age. I do not recommend waiting that long to be conscientious about what you put in your body.

I never counted calories. Now as I am older, I still don't count calories because I eat only fresh, real whole food. Yes, counting calories can be good. For me, I would rather eat my clean diet and not worry about counting calories. More importantly is following the plan in this book to make sure you're eating healthy. Your health unchecked can be like a tsunami, moving very slowly but soon devastating.

Because there are so many books on health, most people will never get time to read them. I have been able to read many and have learned certain things which seem consistent. Especially when reading the information about eating by blood type, you can see all though we are similar with our human body, we are also very different in certain ways. Our daughter Fawn, age four then, was being persuaded to eat something all the other children were eating, and she replied, "But people are different." So true. Just in my circle of friends and family, I found that those of us who are O negative seem to require a little more protein in our weekly diet than those who are not O negative.

Keep in mind that when you try different foods, especially good healthy fruits, vegetables, and fish (and maybe lean meat), don't use another person as your guide. Listen to your own body. Make these changes after you have completed a good detox program. The human body is resilient with some things and sensitive with others.

In your youth, you can eat a diet that is not healthy and survive, and maybe even not get sick. As you get older, your body seems to be more sensitive, and it is important to adjust, continuously listening to your body. A fraction of the time people spend at the doctor's office can be used to make changes to heal themselves by applying the principles in this book.

Water

I started my serious journey to improve my health by reading Deepak Chopra, MD. The most important information I garnered for me was to drink half your body weight in ounces of water per day while drinking most as a flush early in the morning. Perhaps one of his most impressive books *Perfect Health: The Complete Mind Body Guide* was most influential. For me, it was easy because I weighed 160 pounds. So five sixteen-ounce glasses of water per day would do it. If you weigh more and therefore need more water, I recommend staying with five glasses. Just divide the total number of ounces you need by five.

I will talk more about sleep later, but I learned that most people starting in their thirties or forties will wake routinely during the night. Interestingly, most people awake near the 3:30 a.m. time. That was and is true for me. When I would wake during the night (and this is still the case), I drink sixteen ounces of water and go back to bed. When you wake during the night and drink your water, do some stretching while drinking. When I wake in the morning, I drink another glass of water. I also drink one more glass of water before leaving the house. Therefore, if I have one glass of water at lunch and one glass of water at dinner, I have my daily requirement.

It is important to note that if you are sweating a lot, because you are outside in the heat or working which produces sweat, you need more water than this. Also be careful not to drink too much water; it can be fatal. See why balance is so important?

Of course, you may be thinking if I drink half my body weight in ounces of water per day, I will not be able to drink any other liquids. That, of course, is your choice. I chose, when adapting to getting older, to choose the healthier choice. Therefore, I have been drinking only water for many years. I feel good every day, am healthy; and when I go for a medical physical, the doctors are amazed that I am so healthy for my age and have not taken any prescriptions for over a quarter of a century. Actually, I have only taken a prescription when administered in or by the hospital following an injury. I broke my ankle sky diving. I do not take any over-the-counter drugs. Over a quarter of a century ago, when I apparently ate something that did not agree with me and felt bad, I asked my wife what she recommended. She recommended some over-the-counter drug. When I walked from one end of the house to the other to check on that particular drug, I decided to only drink sixteen ounces of water. Within a few minutes, I felt completely better. I realized then that for me, and I would assume many others, the water consumed when taking some pill may be what helps (not the drug). Try it some time.

If you drink half your body weight in ounces of water per day, you may drain in the morning. Your eyes may run. Your nose may run. It is healthy to clean with water.

In the movie *How to Lose a Guy in 10 Days*, Kate Hudson's character, Andie Anderson, made her boyfriend, Matthew McConaughey's character, Ben Barry, blow his nose, and it was clear. Her response was "you are a healthy boy." When it is clear, that is a good flush. Just because your nose runs does not mean you are sick. If there is a color, you are probably sick. Keep plenty of facial tissue, as the flush, especially in the morning, should push fluids from your body. Sneezing is a natural response. Just sneezing does not mean you're sick.

Never hold your water, meaning you should return the water (urinate) at the restroom when you feel the urge. Doctors will let you know that it's not good to restrain yourself from eliminating fluid or waste. If you have the urge during stretching, exercising, or any other time, you should go to the restroom at that time.

God Cures

My legal assistant for almost seventeen years, Annette Forlines, recently gave me two books. I like the way Damon Davis puts it in his book *God Cures: 21 Days to Look Good, Live Great, and Love Well*. He states our digestive system's barrier is like a window screen; the air flows through, but the screen keeps the flies out. Nutrients the body needs are like air. Healing starts from the inside out. Your gut controls everything.

Jack Challem also describes how it works in his book *The Inflammation Syndrome: Your Nutrition Plan for Great Health, Weight Loss, and Pain-Free Living*. Because blood test may not always identify specific immune reaction, you may have to rely on (your own) symptoms in response to specific foods. Nutritionally-oriented physicians recommend strict avoidance of food allergens, and they often suggest that patients follow a rotation diet to reduce the likelihood of new food allergies developing. A rotation diet prohibits eating the same food or foods from the same family, such as dairy, more often than once every four days. Sometimes allergic activity will diminish after several months of avoiding problematic foods.

Smoothies

I have been drinking a fruit smoothie every morning since 2007. My fruit smoothie is made with what fresh fruit I have. I plan so I always have my favorites on hand and at least one green, like kale. If your smoothie is not smooth using the highest setting, you may need a better blender. Some people thought they did not like smoothies because the smoothie was chunky. A good blender is worth the money for those of us who like it completely smooth. I used water but now use almond milk unsweetened to blend, never ice. Very cold food and liquids make digestion more difficult. Add some protein. Almond milk has some protein, and I add some Greek yogurt to get enough protein.

You may soothe your soul and reduce stress with music, meditation, prayer, visualization, long walks, and a positive mental attitude. A fruit smoothie in the morning can contribute to these.

Inflammation

Millions of people suffer from inflammation manifestations, and there are hundreds of drugs marketed to treat them. All of these drugs may mask the most visible symptoms of inflammation. Drugs fail to address the underlying causes of chronic inflammation, and they often have dangerous side effects. People with serious head injuries can throttle up inflammation in the brain that, years later, causes dementia. Drugs may offer a cure that is worse than the disease.

The foods most people now eat do not support the healing process and are in fact proinflammatory and antihealing. The magic of food technologists in adding sugar or salt makes most anything taste good. In our family, we often say cheese will make anything, and I mean anything, taste good.

New Ideas

There are three types of people: healthy, sick, or existing. Follow the information in this book, and be healthy. You deserve to be healthy.

Health experts claim that the more you eat healthy, the more you crave it. That is absolutely true for me. I have been drinking only water for many years and love and crave the taste of water. I do use lemon when dining at restaurants for the slight change of taste. I crave salads and have eaten as many as five in one day. Try it, you may like it (after you do the detox).

Having complete elimination before your morning shower will help in your health journey, and you will be clean and comfortable all day.

Big Family

My siblings are Bill, Jean, Linda, Susan, John, Bonnie, Jennifer, Mark, Ann, and James. I love them dearly. From them and many others, I observed that the decisions we make can overcome genetics in almost every situation, including diet (more later on how science is now proving we can actually change our genes).

Be prepared that most people may not understand your refusal to eat certain foods. It is not necessarily a lonely position, but a position of leadership. Eventually most people will understand the healthy choices.

Be prepared that your love ones may give you bad advice about your diet. I'm sure they mean well, but listen to your own body while making changes to your diet. It took many years to train my family and friends that I would not be eating ice cream and cake at the birthday parties. I have a very large family, and there are birthday parties every month. It was easier for me to just abstain. Some people may get a great result from certain foods, but you may be allergic to those foods.

If you are unable to eliminate in the morning, consume some prunes or unsweetened prune juice before your morning shower. You can train your body to eliminate waste every morning so you can be clean and feel good the entire day. It takes time. You have the rest of your life to train.

Love Life

Being healthy will improve your love life without bad consequences. Drugs always have consequences. Often, they destroy your organs and impair your judgment. People on this diet have found that they function at a level twenty, thirty, or even forty years younger than their counterparts, physically and mentally.

Life expectancy has gone up. We are living longer. But are we living well? Many drugs may help a person live longer, but not well. You can live longer and well, provided you follow the principles in this book. I observed that living a lifestyle with a clean healthy diet, enough sleep, and exercise will help you feel good every day, and you will not suffer the side effects and organ damage resulting from drugs.

Keep in mind that over-the-counter medication and even aspirin are a type of drug. Very few people are on no-drug. Most are on multiple prescriptions. I know people who were given a drug (which did not help) and were then given a second drug to counteract the side effects of the first drug. Are you kidding me? Too many people are taking so many drugs that even the pharmacists question how they can all be working correctly.

If you consume the right foods that have the minerals and vitamins you need, followed by enough sleep and exercise, you have a great chance to be in that tiny percentage, taking *no drugs*.

Proper Nutrition

Proper nutrition can be found in the food you eat, but it takes a desire and determination to make that happen. Eat whole real foods, but if not, start by reading the ingredients on what you are consuming. You may be surprised to know many of the ingredients in numerous foods consumed by the vast majority of the people, at least in this country, cause harm and even cancer. Use the Internet to check the ingredients, especially the ones you cannot pronounce. So many foods cause a host of illnesses, including cancer. Or the easy way is to only eat whole real foods that have no label with ingredients.

Change your thinking. For a snack after dinner, have an apple, orange, or some other piece of fruit. They are sweet and can replace the normal sweet-tooth urge. People tell me "oh that fruit has sugar." It does, but it is different; it is God's sugar. Many people have learned that if you eliminate all processed sugar and the sugar substitutes, the sugar in fruit has no ill effect on them. Amazing!

Artificial Sweeteners (Sugar Substitutes)

Be leery of sugar substitutes. The substitutes, usually chemicals, can have the same effect on some people as the sugar itself, and often worse. When removing processed sugar from your diet, you may also need to remove all sugar substitutes. It is recommended.

It usually takes over three days to get sugar out of your system. It will take between six and eleven days to get artificial sweeteners out of your system. They are not good for you. For a healthy alternative, look at the nutrients in an apple. Have you heard "an apple a day keeps the doctor away?"

According to the United States Department of Agriculture, a large red apple with its skin intact contains about 5 grams of fiber, 13 milligrams of calcium, 239 milligrams of potassium, and 10 milligrams of vitamin C. In fact, a raw apple with skin contains up to 332% more vitamin K, 142% more vitamin A, 115% more vitamin C, 20% more calcium, and up to 19% more potassium than a peeled apple. Apples are also a rich source of polyphenols, which improve digestion, brain function, and blood sugar levels, as well as protect against blood clots, heart disease, and certain cancers. There are so many benefits to eating an apple.

There are about one hundred trillion bacteria cells residing in our bodies. Most are in our intestines. What we eat makes all the difference in how they work to keep us healthy.

My good friend naturopathic Dr. Rachel Smartt says that one year from today, your body will contain nearly 100 percent brand new cells. This means that you literally will be a new you. You hold the power! Rachel says, "One of the greatest ways to catalyst a better health is to navigate better emotions with the things that you choose to think." Every life is a book of secrets, ready to be opened. Anyone who may be moody, irritable, angry, or even irrational may be amazed how a clean diet can remove these.

My good friend Bill Adcox, MD, family medicine practice, recommends nutrition as part of his treatment plan. He was one of the first doctors to include a referral to a nutritionist for my wife. Bill is also a rotary friend who inspires others to get healthy.

Eat supper at least three hours before going to sleep so your digestive system can assimilate the food properly. Any food that is not real food is a bad product and is usually not completely digested and simulated. This forms a residue in the body which is toxic.

There are many varieties of salad. You decide what ingredients you like and make your own salad. When you find a salad you really love, that can be a substitute for the other foods you know you need to eliminate. My personal favorite salad is the Caesar salad with no croutons at Red Lobster restaurant. When you find your favorite salad, if it is at a restaurant, eat there, and think about taking one or two salads with you if affordable. The more you eat the foods you like that are healthy, the more you will enjoy changing.

Restaurants

I have been dining out at restaurants every day since 1974, and most days twice per day. It is less frequent than one in ten years when I eat something that would make me sick. I only eat good food. As I get older, I do notice that even ordering what I consider to be good food may be made with certain spices that do not agree. Therefore, I eliminate those entrées. It is possible to dine out at restaurants and be healthy, but you must be vigilant first in ordering healthy choices and secondly identifying any unwelcome ingredients like certain spices or additives.

Most restaurant owners or managers (and some servers) will tell you if the food choices come from a can, have fat, extra salt, or certain spices. When tasting something that does not agree with you, don't continue eating it for any reason. It is better to pay for something you don't eat rather than get sick. Ameliorate your situation every time.

Water Types

Do not drink distilled water. My experience is limited. But the three people I know who changed to distilled water, two died and one has permanent irreversible damage (with a shortened life expectancy). We believed the water in our county was good for many years. My wife got sick and started consuming a better diet and taking supplements. She did get better, but we also changed her drinking water. About two years after the fact, the county government agency sent a letter saying that the county failed having the required levels of healthy and safe water. Two years after the fact! Incidentally, the time for bringing any claim for injury in this state is two years.

Government employees may not have an adverse reaction to not doing their job, but a private sector is different. We will never trust our regular water supply again. We have ordered verified, filtered spring water since that time. It tastes good, and we feel safe. Do not take your water supply for granted, be safe.

If you can divide the water you need per day into five or six glasses or containers, it is easy to drink one during the night, one when you awake, one before you leave the house; and then if you have one for lunch and one for dinner, you have reached your limit. If six is needed, drink one before going to bed. Getting up during the night to return water (the term I use for urination) is a small price to pay for being healthy. Many of us dehydrate during the night. Sitting to urinate, even for men, is healthier as you are able to fully relax and increase the flow to better empty your bladder.

If you drink this much water, you will need to make a few adjustments. Before you leave your house or any other place, preparing to make a trip, even a short trip, go to the restroom. If you get a massage, even if you don't feel like you need to return water, go to the restroom, sit, close your eyes, and concentrate so you can eliminate before the massage. It only happened one time in my life, but it was very uncomfortable halfway through to have the urge while getting a massage.

Pregnancy

Pregnant women should be concerned about what they eat. The baby is definitely receiving the mother's nutrients and everything else the mother is eating. My granddaughter Maris found that her baby would actually vomit after she consumed greasy chips before breast-feeding her baby Lila. There are numerous similar stories to corroborate how the baby is getting what the mother consumed.

Detox

When preparing to start a detox program, I recommend eating healthy as long as you can before you start. This way, your body will not go into shock from the drastic change. I personally already eliminated the absolutes, those that adversely affected my body, like caffeine, fried food, and most processed sugar. First, you should know that when my friend, who is a doctor, recommended I do the detox, I told him that I was superman and did not need it. But as a strong challenge, I accepted.

Detox programs can range in time usually between four weeks to ten weeks. Mine was six weeks, eating only fruits, vegetables, and fish, with some supplements. While doing the detox, get enough sleep and exercise. At the end of six weeks, I was almost angry, wanting a piece of chicken (or something). However, it changed my thinking. It got my blood sugar where it needed to be. Wow, I was able to be at a table with ten people and be the only one who did not eat bread.

When we are young and resilient, flour and bread products seem to assimilate more easily. As we get older, it seems to overwork our system. Eventually any unhealthy food takes its toll. It was a wonderful change in my life to eliminate all the foods my body did not like, and it gave me the willpower to eat only healthy foods.

Almost ten years later, I heard Dr. Mitra Rae say that "willpower is the function of blood sugar." That was an epiphany for me. I now realized when I was telling people that the detox program changed my thinking. More directly, it had given me willpower because the detox put my blood sugar at the correct level. From that point forward, I not only had willpower regarding what I ate but willpower in every other aspect of my life. I have been reading the Bible and other similar biblical books but was now able to focus better.

I also started with a colon cleanse, recommended by the doctor before the detox. Be ready for opposition. I had close good friends, and family, who would tell me you don't need to be doing that. Some would say, "You are healthy. Why are you doing that?" Others would try different ways to discourage me. Do not listen to them. You will be so happy living a healthy life, and those who discouraged you will eventually see the results. During my lifelong journey of eating better and adapting to healthy choices as I get older, many have voiced opposition.

My minister of music is John Conrad. His wife Donna will respond to something that is gossip or wrong by saying, "I do not receive that." Do not receive criticism for doing what is right. I perhaps had more willpower than others even before the detox; but if you get a challenge or decide you need to be really healthy, get mean, mad even, and do it, whatever it takes.

Our friends at church Nick and Diane Nichols coordinated a church trip. When about thirty people were eating a buffet, I sat next to Diane. I noticed she was the only one not eating dessert (before I stopped desserts). Desserts were included with the meal. Upon inquiring, she replied that the doctor told her she had two choices, go on diabetes medicine or stop desserts. She chose the no-medicine way. This one case was inspiring to me. Let it inspire you too.

I like the statement, "I am from Missouri, the Show Me State." I always say "show me." Sometimes you must show yourself.

Choices

Maybe it is simply two choices. Either you eat healthy, or you don't. Is it easier to say I don't want to spend the time or effort to do a detox? It may be, at the moment, that you can think of the time and effort and pain you will go through at those doctor visits, hospitalizations, very time-consuming commitments or consultations, maybe even surgery, to find and research doctors, that you will realize eating healthy is so much better. Don't forget the financial responsibility and cost, even if you have insurance. Make the real comparison.

Make that decision right now. Go to your refrigerator and food pantry and remove the bad food. If you have other family members who are not on board, you definitely need to detox to get your willpower. It will change your life for the rest of your life.

I believe in prayer. If you believe in prayer, pray for the desire to be healthy. Many years ago, I prayed for God's wisdom. I believe he gave me his wisdom to make better choices than I made in the past. He can do that for you. Ask God for "peace regardless of circumstances" to start this healthy journey now.

Hygiene

Detox includes all areas, including what goes on your skin. In the shower or bath, use a washcloth that actually touches and stimulates every inch of your body. This helps with blood flow and getting things clean. Always use a washcloth. Your hand and soap are no match for a washcloth.

After your shower or bath, completely dry yourself with a towel and then a blow dryer. After your body is completely dry, for dry skin, use 100 percent, pure almond oil. Do not use lotions and soaps that have unnatural ingredients, like perfumes. An exception to this might be between your toes and on your feet, if there is any itching. A good anti-fungal powder is Desenex powder.

During and following your shower or bath, never put anything in your ears smaller than your small finger. Use facial tissue with your small finger to clean your inner ear after a shower. If you must use a Q-tip, use it very gently without pushing it deep in the ear canal, and do not use one more than one time per week. If you have been using a cotton swab regularly, you may need to get your ears cleaning professionally by the ENT. Internet recommends every six months, but usually every ten years is acceptable for most people (provided your ears are not impacted). What goes on your body can be almost as important as what goes in your body.

Pam's Story

My wife, Pam, tells her story in her own words:

Reaching the point of desperation, I prayed for wisdom and called my friend, Dr. Rachel Smartt and asked if she could help me. She told me that plant nutrition is the foundation for great health, cellular detoxification, and gut balancing, and by adding a high concentrated form of fruits, vegetables, and berries in capsule form, it would be the best way to restore and rejuvenate the body. It would "tip" the scale in my favor, making it easier to get back on my feet. It would also fill in the large gap and provide an easier way to get more whole foods in my diet with my struggling effort, low appetite, and drained energy.

She immediately brought me Juice Plus+ and 100 percent clean vegan protein shakes called Complete to my former office (I was no longer able to work) and instructed me in a healthy immune balancing regimen. I also changed my diet. Within three days I was out of bed and began to walk again. Within three weeks my energy was restored, the swelling was virtually gone, I could do pretty much anything I wanted, and I felt I could live again. Rachel, Juice Plus+ and changing my diet literally saved my life! I am so grateful to the healing power of my Lord Jesus Christ, the love and care of Dr. Rachel Smartt, and the life-giving nutrients of Juice Plus.

My wife has shown even when your diagnosis is poor, when you change your diet to healthy whole foods, and in her case adding supplements, you can turn your health to better quickly. Dr. Rachel Smartt authored a book *Modern Day Miracles*, with her daughter Sara Smartt, which has some life-changing ideas on health, hope, resiliency, and transformation. I highly recommend reading this book.

Fasting

Fasting is a delicate subject for me because my entire life I have craved food. Wisdom brought understanding. I believe it is taught in many health books that fasting need not be a multiple-day event. I recognize that fasting can heal people spiritually and mentally, if done correctly. Fasting can be abstaining from something other than food, like television. For me, fasting is done on a daily basis, starting immediately after supper and ending the next day when I have my first food (break the fast, breakfast), which is always a fruit smoothie. This will be a twelve to sixteen-hour period. That is fasting to me. Understand that if food is only going in my body during an eight to twelve-hour period each day, that is fasting. For those who feel the need to fast for a longer time, I will leave that to you.

Prioritize

Prioritize your life, God, family, friends, country, work, leisure, etc. Prioritize your attack to get healthy. To strive for optimum health, use the chronological order listed in this book. You must start with eating right. Once you do that, you will have clarity to choose appropriately. Undoubtedly, that will be to pursue the same order next by making every effort to get enough sleep.

There may be an exception to everything. Some people may prefer a strong exercise program to bring clarity so they can then choose to make the right choices eating. However, my experience has shown eating right will bring the most clarity quickly. Do whatever it takes to live well. By well, I mean feeling good every day, genuinely healthy and taking no drugs.

Adapt to your environment and leisure activities. Recently, in my late sixties, I rode the roller coasters with my grandson Maverick, six feet at age fourteen, super athlete and as rough as anyone. At the end of one ride, the coaster slammed to a stop, which felt like I got a concussion. I could feel my brain slam against the inside of my skull. Maverick then told me he thought he would pass out on the loop. Maybe any age is a good time to reconsider what we volunteer to endure.

Variety

I think we talk to ourselves on a regular basis. Psychiatrists and psychologists know more about this. The vast majority of humans seem to like variety. Variety is the spice of life. Variety is good for investments, food, entertainment, and many other things. However, variety is not good if you are married and lusting for another person. Variety is also not good if you are looking to try foods that you know or suspect are not healthy.

Do some type of detox and change your thinking. You will then be able to use that willpower to make the right choices, not only right choices for food but for everything in life.

Eating by Blood Type

Since the purpose of this book is to save you from reading hundreds of other books, eating by blood type is a consideration. The book I read about eating by blood type was very informative. I only read the section applicable to me, O negative. I actually already eliminated all the foods that were listed as not compatible for my blood type, except one, corn. Corn is not recommended by Dr. Gundry because of the lectins and not recommended for people who may have or be susceptible to diverticulosis. Tomato skin and seeds have lectins.

It will not hurt you to eliminate those foods to see if it helps you. Remember to eliminate them for a length of time sufficient to realize a result. Consider maybe the same time you would use for your detox. People change usually anywhere from four to ten weeks. Since my detox was six weeks, I recommend you eliminate the foods for eight weeks to be sure.

So we don't ignore those fifty years of age or older, when you reach that age, you will be told by your doctors you need a periodic colonoscopy. This is good advice. It is a preventative measure. Select a good reputable doctor by getting a referral from a doctor or repeat patient you trust completely, and there should be no problems. Also if you get a colon cleanse and detox before your first one, it should go smoothly, no pun intended.

Fried

As a youth, I watched women eat fried chicken that was very greasy, who lived into their seventies. The men observed eating these greasy foods seem to die of a heart attack in their fifties or sixties. I do believe they would have lived at least another twenty years eating a healthy diet.

Over the past two decades, I learned in our geographic location that wives may die before husbands. That was a very rare occurrence when I was a child. Even our fresh vegetables no longer have all the nutrients they had when I was young.

It is prudent to live based on current knowledge, acquiring all the health information available, weigh it carefully, and apply it while evaluating the results based on your individual being. It could be confusing to think about the word *balance* when deciding how you eat right. The standard American balance for eating does not apply when striving to be healthy. Most Americans probably think it is acceptable and within the balance to have fried foods maybe once, twice, or three times per week. This is not in the healthy balance. Fried foods are never acceptable because they are harmful to the human body.

One lady had a quadruple bypass heart surgery with 100 percent blockages. She said the surgeon did not recommend any particular diet or any change from the diet she had before the surgery. She had been consuming fried and other greasy foods, caffeine, and processed sugar. When I told her I was surprised, she said the doctor told her it may be genetic, that it was inherited. Upon gently suggesting she may be able to get an upper hand on any problem in the future by changing her diet, she said (and I paraphrase), "Some people will not receive that information."

Fried foods are never healthy for human consumption.

Sugar

Advertising for sugary drinks increased to one billion dollars from 2013 to 2018. Only my wife has known for many years that I had a special time. I called it an epiphany. Being former law enforcement, my home and business have alarms. I've been using this particular alarm at work since we opened the building fourteen years before. This particular day, I forgot the alarm code, which, for the first time, made me think maybe this is not just getting older and forgetful, but maybe a bigger problem.

I am not saying that it wasn't a bigger problem or that eliminating sugar can reverse or cure Alzheimer's or dementia, but I am saying that based on all the health books I read, I remembered processed sugar is bad. I had eliminated all the other so-called bad foods except sugar. I immediately stopped consuming processed sugar. For years now, I have not forgotten the alarm code, not once, not even close.

My friend at church, eight-time consecutive winner as Mr. Olympia, Lee Haney, always says, "Stay away from the poison whites" (white flour, white sugar, white potatoes, and white rice). Processed sugar and processed flour especially are not good for the human body, any human body. Health experts would say they can act as poison. Sugar gives energy, a burst at times, but this energy is usually short-lived. Remember it is not recommended that you eliminate all unhealthy foods at one time. The tapering effect can eliminate the shock to your body and your mind.

Healthy alternatives, for example with white potatoes, can be sweet potatoes. They are much healthier. White flour is in many food products, even including wheat bread (more about wheat later). White flour is difficult to avoid in America. You will need the willpower to avoid it. See the information under the Detox and Willpower sections regarding how to get that willpower. Lee Haney, in his sixties now, continues to eat healthy foods and looks great.

Those who eliminated processed sugar normally find more energy than before. I did. It does not hurt for you to try some of these recommendations. Yes, everybody is different, but some of these foods are not healthy for any person on a long-term basis.

When I totally eliminated processed sugar from my diet, I lost 8 percent of my body weight in the first year. I did not need to lose any weight as I was already slim. My wife insisted I go for a physical. The blood test checked one hundred different items. I am not exaggerating. There are sublevels for many topics. After the results were received and she saw that everything was perfect (within normal range), she then confessed that she thought I had cancer. The next year, I did gain 2 percent that I had lost.

The good news is that eliminating processed sugar from your diet will almost always help you mentally and make you lose weight. The bad news is some people may think you are sick. I would rather people think negatively about me and me be very healthy, as opposed to the opposite. Even if stopping processed sugar only slows the development of an illness, it is worth it.

A person with dementia might live for decades if receiving drug therapy, but is that living well? Our consciousness has no boundaries. We put a man on the moon. God made us. Nothing is impossible with God. Think about these statements. Because our potential is infinite, we dream of all types of achievements. My dream is that most, if not all, Alzheimer's cases will be cured by a change in the diet (and not by a drug, which always has side effects).

We had a speaker at my local rotary club talk to us about dementia and Alzheimer's. I asked following the meeting if any research was being done about the bad effects of processed sugar in that field. She corroborated that there is currently research being done regarding that connection. Stay tuned. I think eliminating sugar in the early stages of realizing memory is slipping can stop or even reverse the disease. Call me crazy, but if you have any memory problems, why not try changing your diet, especially eliminating processed sugar, before using drugs?

Reportedly, dementia is the greatest health threat around the world today. Research now shows that one-third of dementia can be prevented. The good news for the younger population is that if you practice lifelong wellness beginning as early as childhood, the many threats that attack us from middle age onward can be defeated, even dementia.

Staying in high school until at least age fifteen is the biggest single reduction (known currently) to the risk of dementia. Amazing. Are drugs and surgery ever needed? Of course. There are times when they are needed to save a life. This often is when the body's immune system is not strong enough to handle the job and the other times to stop bleeding, reset a broken bone, etc. You are not to ignore or avoid a physician's care when it is needed.

Prior to the coronavirus, COVID, the last epidemic, which still exists, is obesity. We are living in a drug-dependent culture. The average seventy-year-old takes seven (prescription) drugs per day.

Vision

I have noticed an improvement in my vison since eliminating processed sugar from my diet. My prescription has not changed in about two decades. Eyesight is precious, so take no chances. Key ingredients from *Perfect Balance* are drinking half your body weight in ounces of water daily and no processed sugar.

Self-Healing

Research now claims that DNA is dynamic, ever-changing, and totally responsive to a person's lifetime of experience. It is a proven fact that your body can heal itself. Self-healing is possible in almost every situation, even involving disease and illnesses, provided you are making the correct lifestyle choices. The research is amazing, which shows people who change their perspective, change their bodies.

I always wondered why my entire life I had a fond affection for music from my childhood, especially teenage years. Research now shows that songs that were hits when we were between thirteen and twenty-five, we generally bond emotionally for the rest of our lives. Playing this particular music for the particular patient has shown amazing results. One such case is where an Alzheimer's patient was in a vegetative state but when hearing five songs of this music, suddenly woke again, sat up in bed, and started telling a story about his vehicle and first girlfriend, providing perhaps too many details. Parkinson's patients who can barely walk suddenly found their balance and even began to dance to the music.

Caffeine

I was practicing law during the day and in the evening, a detective with the Atlanta police department at the age of thirty-one, working between eighty and ninety hours per week. While driving my detective car on the interstate, I thought I was having a heart attack. I immediately pulled off the interstate to the side so I would not injure anyone else. I was trying to assess the situation, so I did not immediately call for help on the radio. I lay over in the seat, and it subsided. Then I realized it was only heart palpitations.

Since I have been conscientious about how a body reacts to diet, I thought I would test what I had been consuming. Over the next few weeks, I realized I only had heart palpitations when I consumed coffee. I decided to quit coffee.

My friends recommended that I drink decaf coffee. However, when I drank decaf coffee, I had heart palpitations. Good for me, Georgia State University had just completed an experiment, where they were able to determine that the chemicals used to decaf coffee can have the same effect as caffeine in some people. I then knew I was not crazy. Yes, caffeine was the culprit. I would rather quit coffee than go to a doctor to seek drugs that might allow me to continue to drink coffee.

I started a lifelong journey smelling the coffee of others without drinking it. It has been quite pleasurable. The smell of coffee is actually better for me than drinking it. My wife, when drinking coffee, will hold the cup over so I can smell it. She is a sweetheart.

Eventually within a year or so, I realized that I needed to eliminate all caffeine, so I stopped drinking all sodas with caffeine and eating chocolate. Do not get upset. I am not going to ask any woman on this earth to quit eating chocolate. I know better. Eventually, I quit all sodas to eliminate the carbonation, which is not healthy for human consumption. The tapering effect is good for most people, so the body does not go into shock. Start with one food to eliminate and give the body time to show the results.

Bread

White flour, processed flour, and even wheat at times can adversely affect your joints. I should have kept better records of the numerous people who have responded that eliminating white flour from their diet cured their joint pain. There is an exception to just about everything. I'm sure there is an exception to the exception. Regardless, processed white flour is not healthy.

Some people notice that eliminating bread, especially gluten, has cleared their nose and sinus as quickly as a day or two. Although it takes a long time to remove gluten from your system (months), some benefits occur soon.

Obesity

My brother Bill would see a man with a big belly and say that is either a wheat belly and/or a beer belly. My experience has proven him correct. I also know many people who have been obese or overweight, who decided it was time to change, change their diet, and lost all the weight they wanted to lose. Their thinking changed, and the action followed their belief.

Pray for God to open your eyes and mind to a detox for your body and/or the ability to make the definitive decision to be healthy. If you truly believe what God says in his Word, you can do it. If you sincerely and strongly want to do it, you can.

Lectins

Dr. Gundry wrote *The Plant Paradox: The Hidden Dangers in Healthy Foods That Caused Disease and Weight Gain*. This is an in-depth book about lectins in our food. This book is a great read and very helpful.

Just from a clean diet and removing lectins from the diet, Dr. Gundry had patients resolve the following health problems:

- Aching joints
- Acid reflux or heartburn
- Acne
- Age spots, skin tags
- Allergies
- Alopecia
- Anemia
- Arthritis
- Asthma
- Autoimmune diseases (including autoimmune thyroid disease, rheumatoid arthritis, type 1 diabetes, multiple sclerosis, Crohn's, colitis, and lupus)
- Bone loss (including osteopenia and osteoporosis)
- Brain fog
- Cancer
- Canker sores
- Chronic fatigue syndrome
- Chronic pain syndrome
- Colon polyps
- Clamps, tingling, and numbness
- Decline in dental health
- Dementia
- Depression
- Diabetes, prediabetes, insulin resistance
- Exhaustion
- Fat in the stool (due to poor digestion)
- Fibromyalgia

- Gastroesophageal reflux disease, Barrett's esophagus
- Gastrointestinal problems (bloating, pain, gas, constipation, diarrhea)
- Headaches
- Heart disease, coronary artery disease, vascular disease
- Hypertension
- Infertility, irregular menstrual cycle, miscarriage
- Irritability and behavioral changes
- Irritable bowel syndrome
- Low counts of immunoglobulin G, immunoglobulin M, and immunoglobulin A
- Low testosterone
- Low white blood cell count
- Lymphomas, leukemia, multiple myeloma
- Male pattern baldness
- Memory loss
- Migraine headaches
- Nutritional deficiencies due to malabsorption (low iron levels)
- Parkinson's
- Peripheral neuropathy
- Polycystic ovary syndrome
- Skin rashes (including dermatitis herpetiformis, eczema, and psoriasis)
- Slow infant and child growth
- Unexplained bouts of dizziness or ear ringing
- Vitiligo
- Weight loss or weight gain

Ascertain if you are allergic to lectins. My takeaways are that all people are not allergic to lectins, but if you are, you need to avoid those foods with lectins. If you're eating the foods he mentions, which have lectins, and have no problems, you're probably not allergic. If you are very ill and have cleaned your diet according to the recommendations in this book and have not found a remedy, you should read and consider *The Plant Paradox*.

For example, some of the vegetables such as lima beans, which have lectins, can be cooked in a pressure cooker, which removes the lectins. I know this sounds very unusual, and I was surprised to read it. Does not hurt to try. People who are allergic to lectins have been able to cure every disease known to man by removing the lectins from their diet.

My hope is that I can give you enough information to cause a lifestyle change so you can be healthy and happy.

Vegetarian

If you are considering being a vegetarian, you may want to read the book *Forks over Knives: The Plant-Based Way to Help* by T. Colin Campbell and Caldwell Esselstyn. You use forks to eat vegetables and salad and knives to eat meat. Fruit and vegetables are preferred over meat. A seismic revolution in health will not come from appeal, procedure, or operation. It will occur only when the public is endowed with nutritional literacy, the kind of knowledge portrayed in *Forks over Knives.*

For more than 2,800 years, the concept of eating plants in their whole food form has struggled to be heard and adopted as a way of life. Although it is usually defended on ideological ground, recent evidence now proves that this diet produces powerful personal health benefits. What if one simple change could save you from heart disease, diabetes, and cancer? The book has some interesting information, including an x-ray of a man's arteries before changing his diet, which shows one completely clogged artery. There is another x-ray several months later after he was on a vegetarian diet, which shows the artery completely restored.

Your body has the ability to heal itself if it receives the proper nutrition. Of course, adding enough sleep and exercise will speed the recovery even more. I, like many others, have tried the vegetarian diet but felt a little weak. Adding fish, chicken, and turkey restored me to a place of feeling much better. Additionally, I found that for some people, a little lean red meat, usually twice a month, made them feel stronger. My blood type is O, and I subsequently learned that many O-type people seem to need or do better with a little meat. Red meat should be a small portion, fit in your palm, no more than two to four times per month. If you don't need it, stay away from meat, especially red meat.

When I was in my teens, as a truck driver delivering food, I was able to visit two different meat-packing plants. They were making sausage and hotdogs. Think about what would be left to make sausage and hotdogs after you remove the bacon product. It looks like garbage or rubbish to me. In fact, it went down a conveyor belt and fell into large four-foot-high trash cans that needed a forklift to carry the pallets to the next machine that simply added spices to make it sausage. It was clear to see that this garbage later would taste good only because of the spices added.

I was young, invincible, and always believed I was superman. So unfortunately, in my youth, I did rarely eat bacon, sausage, or hotdogs. As I matured and fortunately gained wisdom, I remembered what I saw in the meat-packing plants and stopped eating that garbage. Yes, during my youth, I was sick periodically like everybody else.

Contrary to expensive television commercials, pork is not a healthy food. I will leave it with that and say the experts can debate it as much as they want.

Juicing

I, like many others, pursued the juicing routine for a few years. The time required was draining, and of course, you are losing the fiber from the vegetables being juiced. I now put fresh kale in my fruit smoothie every morning and, of course, eat many fresh vegetables, raw and cooked, daily. I am getting great nutrition without juicing. I am also saving those two hours from start to cleaning.

Minerals

My brother Bill is more of a health enthusiast than I am. He actually started me in the health pursuits: juicing, supplements, liquid minerals, vitamins, good exercises, and focusing on your thinking to reduce stress.

In the late '80s and early '90s, there was a cassette tape—yes, cassette—*Dead Doctors Don't Lie.* The general idea was that you do not need to listen to doctors who are dying in their 50s. It makes sense that you would want to take advice from someone who is healthy and living a long life.

The proposition was to lead you to take liquid minerals. The minerals seemed to help. Ironically, for me, after I had surgery, installing metal plates and screws, the only time I had pain in that area ever was when I consumed the liquid minerals. Not thinking I needed to know the reason for that, I stopped taking the minerals. Also, too many minerals, even without taking liquid minerals, will sometimes let you know you may have too many when you see tiny thin black lines in your fingernails. I still get them occasionally but not near like it was when I consumed liquid minerals.

Supplements and Vitamins

Supplements and vitamins may be needed. Get blood work done by a reputable doctor and lab to determine first if any are needed. If needed, check with a nutritionist to determine which ones would be best. Now there are liquid, looks like paste or glue, in a one-portion packet that seem to be better and work extremely fast. Within a day, for some people, they notice more energy, stamina, and clarity. There are some people who are able to just eat the right food and need no vitamins or supplements.

Dental

The recommended frequency for visits to the dental hygienist is every six months. You should be doing this to keep proper dental hygiene. Medical doctors have developed their thinking (obtained wisdom) in the past two decades and now require clearance from your dentist before you undergo a heart procedure. Does this tell you how important it is to keep healthy teeth and gums? Absolutely. Anything bad from your mouth going down your throat will inevitably cause problems. Very acidic foods and beverages, such as citric juices and soft drinks, are most frequently linked to dental erosion. Hard candy is murder on your teeth.

Many of the health books are now many years old, and ideas have changed, for the better in most part. The healing foods are still fruits and vegetables.

Fruit

Eat fruit first as it digests faster. The best time to eat fruits is first thing in the morning after a glass of water. Eating fruit right after a meal is not a great idea, as it may not be digested properly. The nutrients may not be absorbed properly either. You need to leave a gap of at least thirty minutes between a meal and fruit. However, eating fruit after a meal is better than eating junk food.

Although fruit is good for you, check the quality and ripeness. Don't ever throw a whole piece of fruit in the blender without cutting and checking it. Many look good on the outside but not inside. The outside may need to be addressed. An apple, for example, may have invisible wax covering the outside. A picture is worth a thousand words.

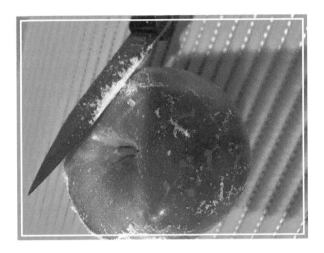

I am not saying that the wax is bad for shipping. It is needed for most fruit, especially apples, because of the time to transport to your local vendor. Just scrape off the wax before eating. The wax actually protects the apple from spoiling. You will learn this when seeing how fast the apple will spoil after having the wax removed.

Two pears (shown below) had wax removed and, within a few minutes, turned brown.

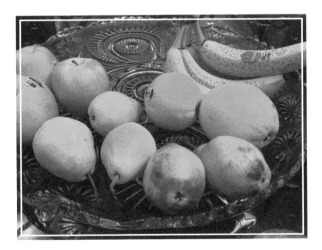

Moderation

Moderation in eating means many different things to many different people. The book *China Study* by T. Colin Campbell and Thomas M. Campbell has one chapter devoted to moderation, and it is titled "Moderation Kills." That is representative of how most Americans talk and act upon moderation.

A quick story about one person who was eating his regular meal of hamburger, fries, and a carbonated caffeine beverage. When I ask what he considered as moderation for that meal, he replied, "You should not have that meal more than once a day." He died in his late forties, and his family members said he always ate a regular diet of fast food.

To live truly healthy, moderation means absolutely no certain foods at any time. Those that have no nutritional value and actually cause harm do not and should not be included in a healthy diet. There is no moderation for those. You know, before I mention them, but if it is something that will not spoil, it is not real.

Since there are so many books on health and fitness, I surmised that readers would rather I read all those books and bring the pertinent information on these topics. Eliminating certain unhealthy foods from your diet is easier when you replace those foods with healthy foods as opposed to abstinence. Many people skip meals because they are avoiding unhealthy foods. Good real whole food will help you replace that void. The elementary school teachers were right. You need three meals a day, and if like me, at least four. Smaller amounts four or even five times per day is better. The metabolism will work better for most people when you eat more often, provided it is the right food.

Your body's healing abilities are almost endless. Following the plan in this book, your body will amaze you. This applies to anyone who wants to move toward perfect health. Not just sick people, but healthy people can actually improve.

Purification of the body starts with eating right and getting enough sleep. Although our body types are different, eating the right foods for you, getting enough sleep, and meditating can help quiet your spirit. This is good. A quiet spirit can help you achieve awareness (more on awareness later).

When eating right, a key ingredient is flushing your intestinal track on a daily basis. Many people find that the morning time is best. All water and maybe some fruit will allow the best flushing.

CHAPTER

Drugs

3

Any silver bullet pill you think is a cure is almost always a trade-off. It will mask the problem or divert your attention and cause more problems, like damage to organs. All drugs, whether over-the-counter, prescription, or street drugs, have side effects. Those side effects can be devastating. If you are willing, you can almost always stop taking all your drugs by changing what you eat. Of course, you must consult a physician depending on what you are already taking, but keep in mind that most physicians are trained to give drugs and/or do surgery. Find a nutritionist first to consult on your nutrition. There have been great strides with many doctors (MDs) who now consider nutrition (your diet) before prescribing drugs—hallelujah.

Many people have told their doctors that they insist on natural remedies, and the doctors acquiesce. The patients are given herbs or referred to naturopathic or holistic doctors. The drugs in this country are killing thousands. It is a silver-bullet drug or pill that is purchased by so many Americans. One poll has it at one-fourth of the population over the age of forty is on some pill. My experience in my area has been probably seventy-five to ninety percent of the population over the age of forty. If you ever pay attention to how many pharmacies there are and how many people visit each pharmacy, you might be amazed.

If a doctor prescribed you a pill and says that it can lower your risk of heart attack by 50% that sounds impressive. However, if your actual risk for heart attack was only 10% then lowering it by 5% is not as meaningful. Could the same risk be lowered by 5% or even more by changing your diet? Almost every time, the answer is yes. Some people decide to start eating a healthy diet after a heart attack or some other life-changing event. Do it as a preventative measure rather than a response.

We need to address the mind at work when taking a pill. The placebo effect has accounted for up to 60 percent of therapeutic effects. Some leading antidepressants have resulted in 50 percent of the positive outcomes due to the placebo effect and only 27 percent to the drugs themselves. Are you digesting this information?

The proceedings of the National Academy of Sciences study in 2014 provide evidence for voluntary activation of one activity link to the autonomic nervous system, immune response. One group training for ten days in meditation, breathing techniques, and exposure to cold had a lower release of proinflammatory chemicals to toxins injected into their bodies. These techniques are now being used to treat patients with autoimmune diseases. When you use the EAGLE plan, you are able to better use these techniques.

Some experts taught that wrist-worn devices that monitor signs of potential disease or stress were good. I actually caution against this if it will cause more stress trying to monitor your every move. Once again, I do not wear any device or count calories because I follow the EAGLE plan and do not need it. And again, we are different, so see what works best for you.

Tao, teaching yoga six to eight classes per week in New York City at the age of ninety-eight, described yoga as union, oneness. Tao says she will teach yoga as long as she can breathe. I plan to work and stay active as long as I can breathe. Staying healthy is the fun part of life. Tao and I both say don't focus on age. It doesn't exist.

Male-Enhancing Drugs

Over the past quarter of a century, I have seen the proliferation of male-enhancing drugs on the market. Most advertisements are actually comical. However, they are devastating in so many cases to so many men.

I am hard-pressed to think of an exception where I know so many men who have been consuming a male-enhancing drug and have developed heart palpitations, heart valve replacement, arrhythmia, or other heart issues. In these cases, my knowledge shows that once it is consumed for a number of years, it is near impossible to correct the heart damage. Some have damage as soon as one year.

Diet Pills

More people than ever are consuming diet pills. There is no shortcut to eating right, getting enough sleep, and exercising. Make a decision to stop the damage to your body and seek professional help if necessary.

I found that people will not receive free advice. But once they pay for it, some of the time, they will listen and apply what they are told. I am amazed at the people who take time to make a doctor's appointment, take off work, drive to the doctor's office, wait who knows how long, and meet with the doctor. An intelligent discussion ensues. Great advice is given. Then these patients ignore the advice and do exactly what they were doing before that lead them to the doctor. They then seek another doctor (I assume seeking to find the magic pill).

Insanity is doing the same thing you have always done and expecting a different result. If you always do what you have always done, you will always get what you always got except as you get older, your body can no longer handle the unhealthy foods as before. You need to adapt to the aging process and continue to move toward a healthier lifestyle.

I pray you find the desire to seek the willpower you need. It is in this book.

Environment

The environment can certainly affect your health. Ticks, which carry Lyme disease; mosquitoes; and other insects can make someone sick regardless of diet. All the more reason to have a clean diet, get enough sleep, and exercise. You will need all the help you can get to give your body the best chance to heal.

Don't inhale hairspray, hair dye, perfume, cologne, strong odors, and other chemicals. Use natural deodorants, like salt-based and others that do not contain aluminum and other harmful ingredients. Use a soap that is natural and does not contain chemicals. Most people only need a tiny amount of shampoo to clean hair. A very small amount of toothpaste, preferably one without chemicals, will clean your teeth sufficiently. Remember to brush your gums as much as your teeth. Massage the gums with your bristles. Be careful with mouthwash, which does not have natural ingredients.

Dishwasher detergent that leaves residue on your dishes can make you sick. We went through a time when I discovered remaining dishwasher detergent particles stuck in the bottom of my glasses (ones I use for water). Although the glasses were upside down on the top rack, the powder remained stuck in the bottom of the glasses. I may have been drinking some of that detergent unknowingly. Although I did not have any ill effects that were known, we switched to a liquid dishwashing detergent that leaves no residue. I was fortunate apparently. I can only imagine the people who may be consuming this who get sick and have no idea why they are sick. Incidentally, it is very difficult to see the white particles in a white ceramic glass or even clear glass. I recommend easily dissolvable gel or liquid detergent. Later, I remembered what seemed like excessive sneezing and saliva during this time. This may have been my body fighting the poison from the powder dishwasher detergent.

There are things that are beyond our control. All the more reason to take control of the things you can. Although information on the Internet changes occasionally, there has been information that the environmental causes of Parkinson's has been welder's fumes, pesticides, and bird feces. Feces of any kind, which reach your mouth, may cause a host of illnesses.

Do not lick envelopes. Use a moist sponge to seal. Do not lick your fingers to separate pages or plastic bags at the grocery store. Be cognizant of everything going in your mouth.

Hold your breath around hairspray, any aerosol, or anything that smells bad. When you inhale these products, you are inhaling chemicals into your lungs, which is never healthy. You need not be paranoid, but be cognizant that you have a choice to eliminate many environmental harms.

If you have a clean home and workplace on a regular basis, you should not need any deodorizers or plug-ins. If you feel compelled to use any, use them sparingly, maybe only a few times a year, the less, the better.

Do not inhale the smoke from candles. If scented candles must be used, use them without lighting. Most jar candles are strong enough to emit a good odor, sometimes for days or weeks after they are closed.

Inside: paint, new carpet, insecticides, or any pest control spray can be bad for inhalation.

Outside: inhaling car fumes, campfires, and any smoke is hazardous to your health.

Men who use hairspray can probably hold their breath and walk away so they are not inhaling any of the spray. Women may need to make more than one trip to try this.

The majority of people who use disinfectants and hand sanitizer seem to be sick as often, if not more, than those who do not. Build your immune system instead. Keeping your immune system in the right place by being healthy will go far beyond disinfectants and hand sanitizers.

Washing your hands before touching your face is a good way to avoid getting sick from germs. Most importantly is following this book to keep a good immune system. Listen to your body.

Technology

Technology involves everything. People are so amazed at my Tesla. It drives itself, has a seventeen-inch monitor, and will certainly protect you with its eleven cameras, motion detectors, and sensors. My rotary friend Phil Hamilton says that it is a computer that thinks it's a car. We are drawn to technology. Be conscientious about how much you use it. I do think the battery-powered car is safer than a fuel-engine vehicle, for us and the environment.

Limit the amount of time your eyes are viewing lighted screens, including your computer, phone, and all other devices. I absolutely love voice texting. This is how I am writing this book. Try not to keep electronic devices too close to your body, especially your head for long periods of time.

There is a documentary on the next step for 5G. It is so interesting. I forwarded the information to all our children to view. Hopefully it will give insights on how we need to limit our exposure. Less exposure to all these devices seems to contribute to a healthier lifestyle.

Stay off your phone and all electronics, especially television, as much as possible. At night, designate one person to receive calls if it is absolutely necessary. Four people in one home need not all have their phones on beside their head during the night. My wife is our designee.

My phone is off and kept in a different room plugged in to power. No television in the bedroom. We agreed before we married. Pam has a television in a different bedroom when she wants to fall asleep to a television. We still love each other. I believe it is essential to good sleep to have no electronic devices where you sleep. It works for me. Remember, listen to your body and do some research.

Television

I never watch the news. It is always bad, with rare exception. My wife gives me snippets periodically, so I am not completely in the dark. However, I like being in the dark as opposed to risking high blood pressure hearing or seeing things that I cannot change. I have friends who have told me after following my decision about avoiding news, especially watching television, they have felt so much less stress.

Alcohol and Tobacco

There is no room for alcohol and tobacco in a healthy diet. You cannot have your cake and eat it too. Are the experts right that a glass of wine per day is healthy? Not exactly. It is the grapes that are healthy, but alcohol is never healthy for the human body. If you do not know that alcohol is unhealthy and impairs judgment, read any of the numerous materials online which show how harmful it is.

Tobacco is similarly harmful. When you try to eliminate alcohol and/or tobacco, remember to replace it with some healthy choice. Quoted from the book *Little-Known Natural Healing Foods and Proven Home Remedies* by Frank W. Cawood, "I'll have a glass of wine and a deadly case of breast cancer to go with my dinner please. It's a ridiculous statement of course but the words are not far from the frightening truth." It says drinking alcohol raises your risk of getting cancer by sometimes as high as 100 percent.

Many people use the Bible as an excuse to drink alcohol. My good friend Dr. Gary Howard who is a double PhD and double masters graduate did a full study of alcohol in the Bible, using the original Hebraic language. Every place in the Bible where Jesus was connected with wine showed that it was one in the bunch. One in the bunch means grapes. The other places for example where Noah was drinking wine was fermented. Obviously, he got drunk from the fermented wine.

The scriptures in the Bible for people to avoid strong drink and wine is often ignored. My accountability partner John Whitworth says that he will not judge anyone for drinking, but he would never drink because he does not want to be a stumbling block to others. I have adopted his view. I also know that alcohol has ruined many lives, led to the death of people too early, and have left many hurting survivors. Alcohol is not good for you!

Charcoal

Charcoal is not good for human consumption. There is a debate about how some small amount of charcoal can be helpful. My observation in life is that charcoal, especially the type that forms on meat when it is grilled, is not healthy. I would not be surprised if one day researchers are able to prove that the black charcoal material on the meat after grilled can be a contributing factor to causing cancer.

The experts now say that every human has cancer cells in their body. It takes two triggers to cause the cancer to grow and become a problem. One factor is stress. Therefore, conceding that almost everyone has some stress, at least there is one more trigger upon which we can focus. The recommendations in this book are where you should focus to eliminate a potential second trigger. Follow the EAGLE plan.

Cures

There are many books about curing cancer by simply changing your diet. Without belaboring the point of diet change, a female German MD in the early 90s wrote a book on how she cured cancer case after case. She first cleaned the diet and allowed at least a couple of months to make sure the impurities from bad food we're gone and replaced the bad food with low-fat cottage cheese and linseed or flaxseed three times a day.

She was curing many types of cancer, maybe not stage four, but many. How hard is it to change your diet to cure cancer? Our politically correct society demands disclosures. I have no personal medical training. I am a person who has observed a lifetime of experiences that prove diet affects everything.

There have been too many times I have experienced people be diagnosed with cancer and not be willing to change their diet—in particular, several with stomach cancer, who were unable or did not have the willpower to stop consuming coffee, sodas, especially diet sodas, sugar, and fried foods. I don't think you need to be a rocket scientist to know that these foods are not helpful to curing stomach cancer. Most people now understand sugar is a cancer feeder. Even the Japanese call canned sodas cancer in a can.

Freedom is available to every person. You have the power and ability to choose the plan in this book to reach the ultimate freedom. The freedom of possibilities will never end as long as you have the good positive thoughts outlined in this book. Reach for the stars. You can actually reach one.

It's not our fault that our parents fed us an unhealthy diet. My mother cooked with Crisco, bacon grease, and other types of lard. She routinely fed us fried foods, hotdogs, and other foods I now call garbage. She loved us dearly—as she would say, greatly—but not armed with the facts about an unhealthy diet.

You have the ability to change that. You can use the information in this book about acquiring willpower, changing your diet, and getting on the right track. Your body also has the fantastic ability of healing itself and quickly. If you have not decided to change your lifestyle to be a healthier person, do it now.

Sun

I have found no better source of vitamin D than the sun. A few minutes of sunshine daily on each side of your body is good. I personally do not wear sunscreen because I am only out a few minutes at a time.

I do not recommend that you avoid sunscreen because we are all different to some degree. However, I believe the adverse effects of the chemicals in the sunscreen are detrimental. The sunshine without sunscreen outweighs any potential risk to me, provided I am only exposed for a few minutes. If you live in an area that does not have sunshine regularly, you may need a vitamin D supplement.

Parkinson's

The cause of Parkinson's disease is still unknown, although there is some evidence for the role of genetics, environmental factors, or a combination of both. It is also possible that there may be more than one cause of the disease. Scientists generally believe that both genetics and environment interact to cause Parkinson's disease in most people who have it.

Currently, there is an enormous amount of research directed at producing more answers about what causes Parkinson's disease and how it might be prevented or cured. When physicians diagnose Parkinson's, they often describe it as idiopathic. This simply means that the cause of the disease is not known.

Scientists estimate that less than 10 percent of cases of Parkinson's disease are primarily due to genetic causes. The most common genetic effect that triggers Parkinson's disease is mutation in a gene called LRRK2. The LRRK2 defect is particularly frequent in families of North African or Jewish descent. Mutations in alpha-synuclein have also been found to trigger Parkinson's, but these are quite rare. In most cases, no primary genetic cause can be found.

Certain environmental factors, such as significant exposure to pesticides or certain heavy metals and repeated head injuries, can increase risk of Parkinson's. Most people do not have a clear environmental cause for their Parkinson's diagnosis, and because many years can pass between exposure to an environmental factor and the appearance of Parkinson's disease symptoms, the connection is often difficult to establish. However, it seems likely that environmental factors do influence the development of Parkinson's, perhaps particularly in people who also have a genetic susceptibility.

There are other things that put an individual at higher risk for developing Parkinson's. The main risk factor is age because Parkinson's disease is most commonly found in adults over the age of fifty (although diagnoses can occur in much younger people). Men also have a higher risk of Parkinson's disease than women. Parkinson's disease often seems to affect Caucasians more than African Americans or Asians. The actual links between any of these factors and Parkinson's disease are not completely understood.

Welders fumes, pesticides, and bird feces at one time were listed as causes of Parkinson's. Regardless, take a super strong approach to getting or staying healthy so your body can have the best opportunity to recover and heal.

Genetics

Understanding how powerful, or not so powerful, genetics can be will help you digest this information. The ability the human brain has to adjust to persevere and survive can help you make choices to override or deal with your genetics. The genetic factor is less important than you may think.

Twins raised by the same parents eating the same food can result with one being a preacher and the other being in prison. What made them make different significant choices? We may never know exactly. However, I maintain that regardless of genetics, if you desire sincerely to be healthy, you can override or deal with your genetics to the point that you can be healthy and happy. What does it hurt for you to eliminate certain foods long enough to see the changes in your body? Not much. The alternative can be devastating and even end your life prematurely. There are only two real main choices in life. Choosing to go through life with God or without God. The next two real practical choices in life is to live a healthy lifestyle or not.

You can improve your genes. A breakthrough sometimes comes from seeing a simple truth hidden behind a tangle of complications. Genes are the most complicated thing in the body. If there is a simple truth behind them, which is you can change your genes, and therefore, you can improve them. You are talking to your genes when you do simple things like eating and moving. That's why recent studies show that people who alter their lifestyle significantly, by eating better, exercising more, and practicing meditation, have changes affecting perhaps five hundred genes.

Immune System

Your immune system can be strengthened by doing the things mentioned in this book. Have you ever thought about the ice swimmers who go swimming in freezing water and do not get sick? Their immune system is healthy.

A complex network of cells, tissues, organs, and the substances they make helps the body fight infections and other diseases. The immune system includes white blood cells and organs and tissues of the lymph system, such as the thymus, spleen, tonsils, lymph nodes, lymph vessels, and bone marrow. The immune system keeps a record of every germ (microbe) it has ever defeated so it can recognize and destroy the microbe quickly if it enters the body again.

The immune system has a vital role. It protects your body from harmful substances, germs, and cell changes that could make you ill. It is made up of various organs, cells, and proteins. As long as your immune system is running smoothly, you don't notice that it's there.

Here are tips to strengthen your immunity naturally.

1. Get enough sleep. Sleep and immunity are closely tied.
2. Eat more whole plant foods.
3. Eat more healthy fats, like olive oil and salmon.
4. Eat more fermented foods, like yogurt and sauerkraut, or take a probiotic supplement.
5. Limit or eliminate processed sugar. Work toward eliminating all processed and artificial sugar.
6. Engage in moderate regular exercise. I recommend three times per week for a minimum of twenty minutes. Jogging, biking, walking, swimming, and hiking are great alternatives to weight training. After age fifty, cardio is recommended three times per week.

7. Stay hydrated. I recommend consuming half your body weight in ounces of water daily.
8. Manage your stress levels. Activities that may help you manage your stress include prayer, meditation, exercise, journaling, yoga, and other mindfulness practices.

Age

Many people focus on age. My father told me it is a number. If a person believes he will be sick, have illnesses, and be on prescription drugs at an any age, he may be right. If a person believes that he will not, he may be right. Actions follow belief!

I have seen too many people who were on prescriptions they said were saving their life to later alter their diet and get off all prescriptions. One reason an exception can exist is when a person waits too long to take corrective actions; it might be too late to get off certain prescriptions. Most prescriptions cause damage over a long period of time. You also know that the drugs can be habit forming, not good.

Future

By the time you read the word *now*, it is in the past. Thinking about it that way, there is no present. We have the past which is beyond our control and the future which is totally in our control. Decide now that your future will be different, a healthier, happier future.

Why is it so hard to make a plan for tomorrow? Usually, it depends on willpower. Read the section on detox to acquire the willpower you need. You may be able to jumpstart your program without doing a detox. If you do try and are unable to stay with the program, do the detox which makes it much easier.

There is a book titled *All I Really Need to Know I Learned in Kindergarten* by Robert Fulghum. Share everything, play fair, don't hit people, and put things back where you found them. These are good, but they don't give you what you need to know to stay healthy so you can do the best job of following these kindergarten recommendations. It must be why we learned the most important part in the third grade. EAGLE!

Some of us litigators used the book *All I Really Need to Know I Learned in Kindergarten* to persuade jurors in closing argument regarding our claim for a person who was injured through no fault of her own. It works well when you're considering a negligence claim. However, this *Perfect Balance* book is focused on you and your health, which affects every aspect of your life.

The vast majority of people, especially Americans, have the full ability to choose what they eat. Perfect health is attainable for most. It is no secret that it starts with what you put in your mouth.

Anything in your body can be changed with the flick of an intention. Have the thought. Act on it, and pursue it. Warts, sores, and other skin blemishes have been seen to appear and disappear with the changing of personalities.

Your body is fluid and all connected. Although we now know we can change the genes in our body, it is good to know your DNA and how you were programmed from birth. Learn your blood type. Research eating by blood type. Adapt to the knowledge you receive. Epigenetics deals with the change to DNA made by everyday experiences, research now shows.

You can actually change your DNA by following the plan in this book. Optimism, great attitude, and not worrying, especially about such things as cancer, can reduce or eliminate any fear, especially about cancer. Experts now say the fear of cancer can be very detrimental. You guessed it. The best attack is having a clean diet every day. And a bonus is that the clean diet not only gives you optimism but works against you getting cancer. It can assuage any fears. Our daughter Candice lets everything roll off. I would always say if we came home and the house was burned to the ground, Candice would say "well, what do we do next."

People mistake instincts, feelings, or cravings for what is right. Use your brain over your emotion or feeling. With the knowledge available to you in this book, you can decide that your brain will control your body. When you receive this and believe it, it will happen.

I know people who said they decided to follow this program regarding diet and did so for about one week. I do not know of any body clock that will be changed in seven days. Most require six weeks and some as long as ten weeks. If you have not achieved it and you have been honest about compliance, proceed forward. It may take you twelve weeks.

Everything you eat, how you sleep, the amount of exercise, how clean you are, and your love for God affect your overall state of balance. Everything you think, say, and do should derive from these. Your overall balance, not just for you individually but for your relationships in the world, can be harmonious. Our daughter Reba is the mediator and human-relations fixer. She has the ability to pursue mending relationships successfully.

Get Enough Sleep

Sleep deprivation is one of the most unrecognized problems in America. Many people have trouble sleeping through the night. Obviously, having a clean diet is very important. Even people who have accomplished the clean diet and exercise on a regular basis may also have trouble sleeping through the night. It is usually a drug or some other thing going in your mouth. I have people tell me they cleaned their diet but still consume coffee. Well, the coffee is probably the culprit. A clean diet means fruit, vegetable, fish, and water. If you are doing this and still have a problem sleeping, keep the regimen for a while, usually six weeks.

In my twenties, when I was working so many hours and in law school, I, like most people, would either find it difficult to slow my brain to go to sleep or awaken during the night with many things on my mind. I discovered that keeping a tablet and pen in my nightstand could solve the problem. When I would wake with something pressing on my mind, I could actually open the nightstand drawer, remove the tablet and pen, write what was on my mind without even opening my eyes. The next morning, on occasion, it was difficult to read my own writing; however 99 percent of the time, I was able to read it. This allowed me to go back to sleep, knowing that I would not forget it in the morning. Even things I believed to be unimportant could also be noted to allow me to clear my brain. This allowed me to get a good night's sleep.

I have read authors who say that you cannot catch up on lost sleep. I respectfully disagree. If you need eight hours' sleep per night and two nights during the week you get six hours, if you sleep in Saturday morning to three or four extra hours, it can be very helpful. You may not have 100 percent on your required sleep, but you will hopefully find what I did that it felt like you had caught up on your sleep. Remember positive thinking goes a long way. All of this may be realized because of applying the EAGLE.

The key to getting enough sleep for me is keeping the bedroom completely dark with no lights. This means no illuminated clock, TV off button (when we travel), or any other light whatsoever. My wife goes to bed with the television on and, like most people, does not sleep through the night. She wakes and may be awake for hours.

Even the healthiest people can awaken during the night and not go immediately back to sleep. One thing that can easily be tried is to lie there in the bed very still with no light whatsoever and with a slight hum from a fan or noise machine, pray or meditate to calm your mind; and surprisingly, your next thought may be awakening in the morning.

To help you sleep, consider some peaceful low noise or a fan. The fan which emits a low-level hum is soothing to most people and helps them sleep. A sound machine also is an option. The one with several different noises, including ocean waves, white noise, and running water have helped many sleep. Some even like the thunderstorm noise.

When writing this book, I would write buzz words on the tablet on my nightstand beside the bed so I could sleep. The next morning, I was able to use the buzz words to complete many paragraphs of what I intended to write. You may think of ways to develop more options to improve your sleep.

My experience in life has been that people who start reading a book, watch television, or have any device with a light like a computer, or even the light from your radio clock, do not go back to sleep for some time.

If you try these simple ideas and it does not solve your problem, remember it's probably because of diet. Diet is number one for a reason. If you need to be able to see your clock during the night, have a lighted clock so you need not have an overhead light. Also after viewing the clock, turn it away from you so if you do wake during the night, you will not see the light to cause any stimulation.

When using eye cover to help you sleep, make sure it is soft and comfortable. You may also want to have the thickness needed to block the light. There's also one that is inexpensive but has a piece on each side of your nose to block the light from the bottom. We need total darkness for the best sleep.

My wife and I have been on many cruises around the world, and only one time did we try an interior cabin. It was some of the best sleep I ever had, absolutely no light. We always get a balcony because it is more fun and enjoyable because my diet allows for good sleep without complete darkness.

Your body is made to sleep while it is dark outside. Keep it dark inside as well for better sleep. During the night, most people move, turn, and change positions. I think this is a good natural part of being healthy. You may understand how people in nursing homes or even hospitals for longer than a few days will get bedsores, if not moved.

You can have good sleep when you are changing positions during the night. Sounding like a broken record, if you have a truly clean diet, you should get good sleep. If you are on this truly clean diet and not getting good sleep, maybe you're not allowing enough time in the bed. Some people need nine to ten hours per night. This could be ten hours in the bed with eight hours' sleep.

The experts say you need eight hours sleep per night. Teenagers need maybe ten or eleven hours. When teenagers sleep twelve hours, it may be that they really need it. When you sleep for six hours a night and say you feel good and that's all you need, you may be wrong. Although you may feel good now, you may be shortening your life by years. Usually we do not know more than the experts. One exception is that the mainstream MDs that do not follow a nutrition platform before administering drugs and surgery should be followed very carefully. Think outside the box and adapt. If you're truly on a clean diet and after ten hours in the bed, you are not getting enough good sleep, you may have a serious problem and need to see a physician.

I do not recommend earplugs while you sleep because they seem to interfere with equilibrium after a long period of time, like sleeping eight hours. I recommend turning the fan to a higher setting if there are noises that need to be blocked. You may also use the sound machine at a higher volume. Find something that gives you a soothing feeling to drown out the unwanted noises. Never use a television or any other electrical device to help you sleep. The only time I use earplugs these days is just for any speaker or noise, which usually lasts less than an hour. You should be able to understand the speaker while wearing earplugs. My whole life, I've been hearing about people getting old and become hard of hearing. I have actually experienced more sensitive hearing the older I get. I do believe that is directly in response to the clean diet and getting it cleaner as I get older.

If you have congestion when you go to sleep and will need to clear your throat or nose, keep tissues on the nightstand or even a small trashcan beside your bed. Keep a lined trashcan or cup beside your bed so if you need to spit, you can do so without opening your eyes or leaving the bed. This way, you will not need to leave the bed to go to the restroom. Do not be embarrassed. This is your life and health. Do what it takes to stay healthy. If you don't take care for yourself, you will not be able to take care of anybody else.

If you wake when you change positions during the night, lie still, quiet, and keep the room dark so you can return to sleep. If the back of your head gets hot lying on the pillow, move slightly to another spot on the pillow that is cool. It is easier for most people to sleep when the room is cool and the back of their head and neck are cool.

Options for sleepwear should be considered: cotton, flannel, booty socks, and even sleeping nude. Sheets may be cotton, silk, flannel. Find what works best for you. All these options make a difference if you are not sleeping. During the night, it may change.

Find the right mattress for you. Even an investment in a motorized mattress can be life-saving. Different pillows make a difference. Do what you need to do to accomplish sleeping well.

People can laugh; but it is true that turkey, especially the real lean turkey breast, makes many people sleep straight through the night, even eight hours before they wake. The tryptophan works on so many people. You do not need to wait until Thanksgiving to have that good sleep without drugs. Of course, having a good clean diet all around will help the turkey do its job.

Interestingly, you should wash your hands before going to bed. From the mint flavor on your floss that is now on your fingertips or anything else you may have touched, most people touch their face many times during the night. Washing can certainly prevent eye irritation.

Every morning when you wake, stretch. My favorite is to put your hands behind your head and arch your back as far as you can, like a cat. Stretch every muscle you can with your eyes still closed. If you must return water first, return to bed and do the stretches. You will feel better as you start your day.

Sleep is the second most important focus for physical heath in your life. The first obviously is diet. Ironically, birds and other animals can wake you in the morning. To avoid this, turn your fan or sound machine to a higher level to block noises that may wake you. If animals in your home bother you, only you can remedy that.

You can train your body to awaken at a certain time, but you must go to bed at a certain time for your body to get enough sleep to do that. You should find that you need a certain average of hours per night to feel good. If you sleep ten or eleven hours Saturday morning and feel great, you probably needed it. If you feel tired and you're following the recommended plan in this book strictly, then see a doctor.

Deepak Chopra says a still, undisturbed state of awareness is whole mind. I found that state each morning in the quiet when I stretch, also each time I visit a restroom where it is quiet.

Many years ago, our daughter Lauren would tell us when she was awake with her eyes open that she was thinking of nothing. I often questioned that. Lauren made straight As, had common sense, and was an all-around good God-loving girl. Later in life, I learned this is a good thing. It is normally recommended for the first awakening moments before you get out of bed. There is no intervening part to block your awareness. You can expand these few seconds into a conscience experience. This works especially well for me because I have no alarm clock. My body clock allows me to know how many hours of sleep I need so when I go to bed, I know what time I will wake. If there is a priority the next morning when I have been up late the night before, I may set the clock, but I usually awaken before it alarms.

After drinking water during the night, train your body to go back to sleep. This is done by lying still, but relaxing; and if you have the urge to return water, go to the restroom at that time. Each time returning to the bed, lie still in a relaxed state with all the conditions that promote sleep like keeping the room dark with no lights and no sound, or sound that you prefer like the hum of a fan or sound machine. If your mind races when you try to do this, continue doing it, and eventually you will train yourself to relax. Your body also needs several of these relaxations during each day.

Benjamin Franklin's premise was that early to bed, early to rise makes a man healthy, wealthy, and wise. Sleep is very important, but if you're not eating right, it may be very difficult to get the good sleep you need. As you sleep during the night, keep an open mind about staying comfortable. This may mean changing clothes during the night. Keep the anticipated clothes close by so it is easy to change. Some people get warm being in bed a short time but then get cold later during the night. Some may need no clothes but need them before dawn. A comforter is too much for many, including me. It absolutely makes me too hot. Many people like a sheet over them even when they don't need it for warmth; obviously it does not offer much warmth. Plan your attack before you go to bed. Plan appropriately, and you will succeed getting a goodnight's sleep. I keep my clothes on the bed for easy access during the night if I should get cold.

Exercise

I have been exercising on average three times per week since the age of thirteen. I have modified continuously but stayed the course because it was a habit. In order to establish a habit of exercising, I recommend starting with a routine that is so easy you can do it if you are sick. The key is to do it a few times per week every week so it becomes a habit. Once it is a habit you can increase your reps, sets, and routine.

When exercising, stretching, and lifting weights, I close my eyes. It helps me. People are different, so see what works best for you. I work out (and stretching during my workout) with my favorite music, but complete silence when stretching each morning. The variety is good for me.

I have no need to know why it is easier and feels better for me to close my eyes. It works for me. Explore the possibilities. Find something that makes it easy enough for you to form that habit of exercising on a regular basis.

When lifting weights, do not go over eight reps if you are building strength. Usually, three sets are recommended. If you are seeking to lose weight, do more than eight reps, usually fifteen. Usually, three sets are recommended.

As you get older, use dumbbells instead of free weights, palms down. Nautilus is good.

So many people have low back problems. If the low back pain or stiffness is from a pulled muscle, you may be able to benefit from a simple stretch. Dr. Michael Hartpence has been prescribing stretching for many years. I witnessed him testify in a jury trial for me where he explained how this all fits together. He will tell you that diet, sleep, exercise, and stretching are vital to good health.

Swimming is one of the best exercises on the planet. If your body prevents any exercise, do what you can until you are able to do more. Set a goal and persevere. I had an injury where my back muscles in the lumbar region were strained. Throughout the years, occasionally I was unable to stand straight. In the mid-90s, Dr. John Giovanelli showed me a stretch, which eliminated that problem. I have been doing that stretch every morning and every night since the mid-90s. I'll do it in the morning while I am drinking my fruit smoothie so it cost me no time, and I do it in the evening while I am flossing my teeth so it cost me no time. If it works, do it. Think outside the box. Incidentally, I have shared this particular stretch with numerous people, most of whom told me that it was a lifesaver and their problem was solved.

There's an endless variety for the treadmill. I recommend starting with something easy for twenty minutes three times per week until you are in the habit. After you have formed a habit and feel like you can increase, the options are endless. Just by way of example, one I have used is to walk the first two minutes at 3.5 on the treadmill, run at 5.5 for thirty seconds, and then return to 3.5. The second set can be increased to 6.5 at thirty seconds. Three sets with a maximum of five sets seem to work well if you are healthy. After three sets, walk the balance of your time at 3.5 to 4.0. Don't rush. It is better to do less without rushing than to rush your exercising and harm your body. Slow is better.

Breaking the Chains

You can make a breakthrough with your health when you realize that billions of dollars are spent to cure the body of many illnesses, diseases, and miseries. Attack the problem seriously. Every bite of food you eat alters your daily metabolism, electrolyte balance, and proportion of fat to muscle. Every minute of sleep you get heals and refreshes your body. It rejuvenates. Every time you exercise, you are putting money in the bank, becoming stronger, and increasing mobility such as range of motion. Every hour of total inactivity creates muscle atrophy.

You need gravity and resistance when exercising. Don't fight it, welcome it. When you look at exercise not as a chore, for example, but as a way of increasing your focus and energy, you have created a new interpretation. Now the burn of your muscles on the stair master and the wind you feel after running a mile are positive things, not reasons for distress. This changes your body's experience. I reached this realization before reading health books. I believe it occurred because of the plan outlined in this book, EAGLE.

If you cannot jog or run, start by walking. Even on the treadmill, you can walk. Try to increase your walking until you are able to sweat at twenty minutes. You need to stay active to be healthy. When you are young, if you choose to believe "no pain, no gain" and that mentality works for you, use it. However, as you get older, it is rare when that system works. You should receive more from your exercise than your input.

It is recommended that you never exercise on a regular basis approaching 100 percent of your capacity. I remember ending my strongest year at age forty. When bench-pressing my max, I saw stars. It is not just in the cartoons—it is real if you exert yourself to that extreme. I stopped before injuring myself. When you get older, it should be a tapering effect to no more than 50 percent of your maximum capacity. As you get older, a continued tapering effect is normal.

At the first sign of overexertion, stop exercising, give yourself a few minutes of walking around to let your system cool down by stages, and then rest for another few minutes until your heart and breathing are back to normal. During your exercise program, continue to breathe freely. If you feel you're not getting enough air through your nostrils, open your mouth. Therefore, it is recommended that most people do not hold their breath.

Never strain or push your body. Never bounce when you are in a position or pose. Focus on your body as you stretch. Sometimes it is beneficial to stop or lessen the stretch and then resume the stretch after a small break.

Exercise on a flat, non-slippery surface, such as carpet, rug, blanket, exercise mat, or other semisoft surface. Remember that you are listening to your body but also applying knowledge from this plan. You should be adapting to what works best for you.

Stretching

All stretching outlined can be done with no gym or weights. The human body can benefit from stretching every morning and evening and even other times during the day. Especially every morning is needed as you get older. I did stretching every morning for many years before I learned what I was doing was actually yoga. Find a routine that is easy to start, and eventually, it will be a habit.

Interestingly, I learned that stretching your neck muscles can change your teeth and jaw. My teeth were straight my entire life, and I never needed braces. After having a crick in my neck muscle, I decided to add another stretch to my morning routine. The stretch involved pulling my neck (using my neck muscles) as far as it would go in several directions. Within several months, my teeth became crooked. A trip to the endodontist proved very helpful, and we began a regimen of straightening, using the clear trays. After a year, my teeth were straight again. I now use the teeth trays in the morning while stretching.

If something changes following you doing something you know is right, seek a remedy. Don't stop doing what you know is right. The crick in my neck never returned. That has been over seven years ago.

Many of my stretches look like a cat. We all know cats are some of the most flexible and versatile physically. Start every new stretch and every physical exertion gently until you are convinced you can go farther.

Stretch 1

I start extended stretching with sitting on the floor with my legs apart as far as they will go, toes down for fifteen seconds and toes up for fifteen seconds. I stretch my neck in all directions at the end of each stretch. Hold head up, turn head right as far as it can go, turn head left as far as it can go. Hold head down and repeat turning head. Do your neck exercises (during the stretch) at the end of each stretch. You may want to start this with your back against a chair or wall for support.

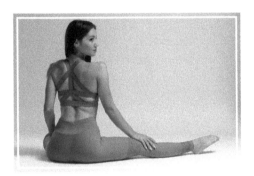

Stretch 2

Crouch with your torso on your thighs and upper body hanging over your knees as far as it will go for at least thirty seconds. Relax your arms beside your legs, usually with hands on the floor. This will allow for easier transition into the next stretch.

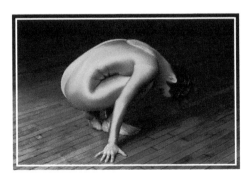

Stretch 3

On your knees with your shins flat on the floor with your toes pointed backward. Now straighten your upper body with your spine completely straight going up toward the ceiling for thirty seconds.

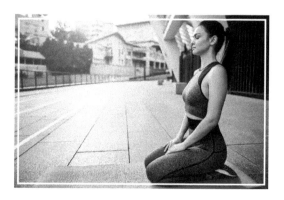

Stretch 4

Put your body on your thighs leaning forward as far forward as possible for fifteen to thirty seconds. With your forearms flat on the floor with your elbows touching your knees, preferably on carpet or a mat, lean your head forward as far as it will go. Hold for fifteen seconds, and raise your head as high as it will go for fifteen seconds, followed by routine neck stretches.

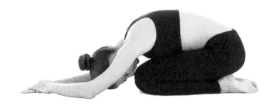

The time depends on when you may hear a slight pop, which is your body helping your alignment. I hear it often at five to eight seconds, but occasionally it may be twenty-two to twenty-five seconds. Try going longer to see if you have an alignment occur after thirty seconds.

Stretch 5

With your shin still flat on the floor, with your toes pointed behind you, lean down, and reach your hands as far forward as possible with your palms down flat on the floor. Hold this for thirty seconds. Then without moving, do your neck exercises.

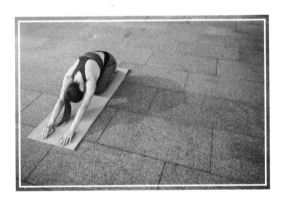

Stretch 6

With your knees still on the floor, raise your body up, reach out, and place your knuckles on the floor, with your triceps (upper arm) parallel with your back (and floor). Your torso is parallel with the floor. This position works better with your back relaxed and your head down.

Use the following position shown in the background first. If your back is strong enough, you can try the position in the foreground, with knees off the floor. The position in the background is sufficient for most people. You may bring your knees forward until it is easy and most comfortable for you. Knees under your hips is an easier position.

This can be thirty seconds. For many people, it may take thirty seconds to reach the point where you hear a sound like a pop, which is your spine going into alignment.

For an easy start, you can do the position in the background with your knees under your hips.

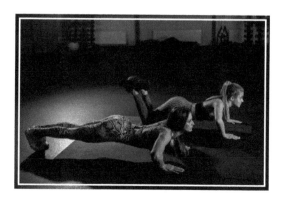

Stretch 7

While still on your knees, hold your arms straight pushing downward to raise your back like a cat, with your knuckles on the floor, close to your knees. Put your arms in front, keeping them straight from the shoulders to the floor. Arch your back as high as you can for thirty seconds. Don't forget your neck exercises (during the stretch) at the end of each stretch. The position in the photo may be used, but the position described above offers a tighter arch.

Try a longer period to see if the popping in your spine or ears will cause you to feel better. Occasionally, you need to stretch longer to have these areas return to normal.

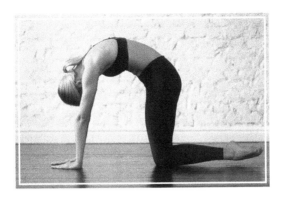

Get in the crouch position again with your chest resting on your thighs and your arms around your knees, with your palms flat on the floor, almost under your knees for fifteen seconds. Without moving, raise your hands with only your fingertips and thumb touching the floor so your palm is raised upward.

When bending your head down, do not force it to your chest.

Stretch 8

Do a plank or heel raise. The plank is done with your body straight, in the push-up position, with your toes and forearms on the floor. You should start with only a few seconds to determine that you will not have a spine problem. In full disclosure, if you had a prior back injury problem, you may want to consult a physician or physical trainer.

The heel raise is usually easier than the plank. Heel raise is lying prone on your back with your heels raised one to two inches off the floor. Do not use your hands or arms to help you keep your heels off the floor. They may be resting gently on your chest, stomach, or floor.

With the planks, see if you can work your way up to two minutes. With the heel raise, you may try the same or do sets of one minute each. Between each heel raise or plank, it is recommended that you do a stretch lying prone on your back with your toes pointed upward and your fingertips stretched, pointing as far over your head as you can do. Do this for fifteen to thirty seconds and then the same with your toes pointed downward, away from your body, for the same length of time.

While lying in the prone position on your back stretching, when you can, continue to stretch even further. Just because you start at a particular position, often you are able to stretch further during the stretch. This is good. Watch a cat, which is one of the most flexible animals in the world. Stretching is very beneficial.

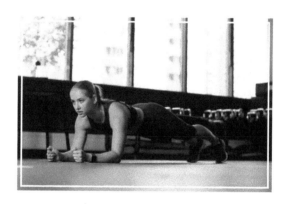

Stretch 9

Lying on your back, pull your knees up on your chest and your arms over your knees, holding hands and pulling your knees as far down to your chest as comfortable. With right arm over your right knee, grab your left wrist. Pull your knees to your chest for fifteen seconds. Then repeat fifteen seconds with left arm over your left knee, holding your right wrist. If you cannot reach that far over your knees, then you may need to hold your knees with your hands, right hand on right knee and left hand on left knee.

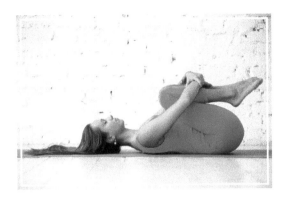

Upon completing this part, to achieve extra flexibility, you can move your feet back and forth with one on top of the other quickly. This usually leads to some popping. Make sure you do it gently until you are accustomed to going beyond the gentle phase.

Upon releasing your knees, rotate your feet, with your knees still high in the air. Rotate them outward and then inward for just a few seconds each. The popping in your spine and ears usually means your spine is being properly aligned, and your ears are being cleared where you can hear better. Both of these may not occur until after the detox (of usually at least six weeks) and exercising properly. The stretching recommended for fifteen seconds may need to be increased to thirty or even sixty seconds to achieve these results.

Stretch 10

Upon completing the sets, get in the crouched position again with your chest on your knees and hands on the floor, with your arms going beside your knees. I actually hear the slight popping throughout my stretching. Remember to do your neck stretching at the end of every stretch mentioned. This entire process can be done between twenty and thirty minutes depending on the number of sets. Fifteen to twenty minutes is a good minimum stretching session, always after you have consumed sixteen ounces of water.

This series of stretching is done every morning. Do this even before your full workout days (three days per week). With your eyes closed, you can count one 1,000, two 1,000, and so on to know your timing. At the end of each stretch, regardless of how many seconds, if it feels really good, stay in that stretch for a while. After all your stretching, if you have trouble going to the restroom before your morning shower, do the pushing up like a cat exercise (position 7) in extra sets or until you feel the urge to eliminate.

Experiencing a slight popping noise during stretching, as well as all other workouts, is usually a sign that it is helping. However, people with prior damage or injuries should consult an expert. An expert in this case is usually an MD, like an orthopedist.

For clarification, after each stretch, while staying in that position, tilt your head backward as far as you can, which stretches your neck as far as it will go. While holding this position turn your head to the left as far as it will go and then the right as far as it will go. Bring your head tilted downward with your chin closer to your chest, turn your head as far left as it will go and then as far right as it will go.

We have heard all our lives how important posture can be. It is important. However, if you have a strain or injury in your low back, an erect posture may actually aggravate your injury to hold yourself erect for long periods of time. I cannot count the number of men I know over the age of forty who have low back pain, almost always in the lumbar, L4-5. That is the point in your back where the most pressure is applied when bending and pivoting.

A clean diet as discussed in this book may not cure your problem, but why not try the clean diet before drugs and surgery? Even if your situation requires surgery, the clean diet will help you with a faster, easier, and better recovery.

It is a good idea to stretch throughout the day. Even while at work, plan to stretch. If you have a desk job, plan to get up move away from your desk and do some light stretching if only for a few minutes. If fifteen seconds feels too short, extend the time, never less than fifteen seconds. If thirty seconds feels too short, extend the time. If reaching a fifteen or thirty-second time and you start to yawn, continue stretching until you completely finish your yawn.

The times listed for stretching represents one set. This should be a minimum of one set. The older we get, we sometimes sound like the rice crispy cereal—snap, crackle, pop—but that is better than the alternative. While stretching in the bed, roll around stretching; have fun, act like a kid. Decide it will be fun. It certainly is enjoyable.

Do not interrupt, block, or prevent a sneeze, burp, yawn (and even a cough if you're not sick). This is a natural response of your body and often to eliminate something not needed. There is plenty of medical advice about yawning or excessive yawning (whatever that is), but that advice is negative. I believe it can be a sign of needing more oxygen but can also be because a person is bored. If you are otherwise healthy, yawning can properly stretch your muscles and give you more oxygen.

You can train your body to eliminate waste every morning so you can be clean the entire day. It does take time. You have the rest of your life to train your body.

Weight Training

Since I continued to get stronger every year until age forty-one, I lifted free weights. Reaching my max at age forty, I weighed 167 and was bench-pressing 345, no steroids or any substances! The increasing effect going to age forty-one reversed and declined each few years thereafter. I reached the point where I realized that stretching was more important than heavy free weights. I eventually stopped heavy free weights and went to nautilus weights and dumbbells. Stretching is essential in your workouts and any exercise routine.

Lifting weights is good for you. When you are younger and you have a routine for example three days per week, after a year or two for most people, it is good to take a break. I would not lift any weights on vacation for a week or two, come back to the gym, and actually be stronger. Your body routinely needs rest.

As you get older and you're maintaining, the same break may not work for cardio. Consistency is good as you get older, especially for cardio. Do cardio three times per week.

There are many styles of exercising. Don't think you must choose one. Make it a variety of styles that suit you. For example, the experts for many years said not to hold your breath while lifting weights. I have been holding my breath on particular lifts my entire life. So it is proof for me that it has worked, and very well.

During the five years I worked between eighty and ninety hours every week, there was little time allocated to exercise. However, I was young, resilient, and followed a decent diet, eating many healthy foods. As you age, it is imperative that you adapt and make every effort to put diet first.

If skipping or reducing what you do, reduce the weights before you reduce your stretching. Stretching is more important.

Cardio

Also, when you reach fifty years of age, your doctor will recommend, if not before, a stress test. This is good advice. Do you want to learn if you should be doing cardio three days per week? This test will show you.

Again, there are so many books written about this type of exercise (cardio). I have gleaned nuggets which show to my understanding that you should always make it at least three days per week for valid cardio exercise. This means to be valid according to the experts, you should be sweating after the first twenty minutes.

I always believed that I was Superman. However, my first stress test at age fifty showed that I did not have optimum health, like Superman. Even though I was still healthy, I decided to add running and more jogging to my routine. I started with twenty minutes on the treadmill, did that for many years before increasing to twenty-five minutes. Then within probably a year, I went to thirty minutes and another year thirty-five minutes. I've been doing thirty-five minutes on the treadmill following my regular weight and stretching exercises for many years. It keeps me healthy and happy.

I chose the treadmill in my home so I can choose my music, my temperature, avoid insects, avoid traffic like noisy, smelly dangerous vehicles, and especially dogs that might chase (and bite) you. I understand being outside in the fresh air has an advantage. I'll do it when I am not jogging. This way, I always complete my thirty-five minutes uninterrupted. You choose. I can actually read the entire thirty-five minutes.

Cardio exercise is good at any age. Start as soon as you can. On a personal note, I ran track in high school, was actually very good. I ran varsity track in the ninth grade. However, upon graduating high school and working sixty to eighty hours per week, I stopped running. There are many reasons to avoid exercising. Do everything in your power to avoid those reasons and make it happen.

Colonoscopy

Colonoscopy is also recommended at age fifty. In full disclosure, I should let you know my first colonoscopy, even though I have a clean diet, was an unpleasant experience. An anesthesiologist gave me some medication that allowed me to wake during the middle of the colonoscopy. I am now having the conversation with the doctor, who is saying, "Look, everything looks so pink. That's good." I was certainly glad to hear that, but I definitely wanted to be asleep during the entire process. I asked a good friend David Anders, MD, at church, who is very healthy, who he used. I started using his doctor and smooth sailing all the way. Dr. Anders is highly respected in our community.

You may never change your eating habits unless you bring healthy food into the house. This does not happen by chance. Decide on a plan of what healthy foods you are willing to try. Make a note, take it with you to the store, put that food in your shopping cart, and bring it home. This is the beginning for most people.

Wash Your Hands   6

"Wash your hands" means all cleanliness that is needed to stay healthy. If your dental hygiene leaves any odor, consider a tongue scraper. Most people are shocked to find the food that can be removed from your tongue after brushing your teeth. In addition to brushing, floss your teeth every night before bed and water irrigate preferably to be certain there's no food in your teeth or gums when you go to bed.

Always close the lid to the toilet before flushing. The Internet has videos showing the spray from flushing and even sneezing that can go as far as fifteen feet. Never brush your teeth while on the toilet. Please watch this video once. That should do it. Train your body to eliminate before your morning shower so you will be clean the whole day. Washing your hands before touching your face is a good way to avoid getting sick from germs. Most importantly is following this book to keep a good immune system. Listen to your body for food response, not cravings.

Animals

There are materials that animals have proven to be a benefit, maybe even a tremendous benefit, to some people. Those people might be people who live alone, in a nursing-home-type environment, or people with certain disabilities. However, there are numerous people who have problems because of animals. Allergies, of course, can make people sick. Animals are not always clean. When people kiss an animal around their mouth, it is risky. Animals put their mouths in places that carry diseases. They shed and have dander that is unhealthy when inhaled.

There are many places your mouth should never touch. Those oral contacts should never be animals, and be careful with human body parts. You are what you eat, and you are what gets inside your mouth. See detox for details on living clean.

Routine

For almost a quarter of a century, I have been waking in the morning without an alarm clock. A good routine is to wake without an alarm clock, return water, and eliminate if possible. Drink a glass of water, preferably sixteen ounces, never cold. Do your daily stretches. And remember to use your balanced breathing, always in silence, which allows for meditation or prayer. If it is your day for exercise (workout), follow with exercise.

Now it is time for breakfast. I have been consuming a fruit smoothie for about fifteen years, which provides the fruits and some vegetables I need for that day in an easy smooth drink. Always follow by brushing your teeth, especially if you have blueberries. They will stain your teeth like coffee if not removed quickly. One secret is to drink your smoothie while wearing any teeth trays so your teeth do not stain. Try using a tongue scraper to see if any white film is on your tongue. After cleaning your diet, you will normally see no film. If it persists after truly cleaning your diet, there may be another problem.

Bath or shower time. I am a shower person and enjoy warm water. The warm water is actually recommended by the health enthusiast. However, as my friend and partner Michael Brennan says, "Use cold water on your head when shampooing because it retards hair loss." The cold water is not that bad. You can actually stand away from the shower water and lean over with only your head in the cool or cold water.

Now it is time to reconnect with nature.

It is recommended that lunch be your largest meal of the day. I confess I struggle with this one. I like every meal to be a big one. Carve out at least five minutes after each meal of the day for silence. If you need, you may always go to a restroom and hopefully sit in silence. It may sound odd, but it is important.

As we males age, our urination slows, sometimes significantly. I have friends who opted for the Roto-Rooter to open the canal. Some experienced ill side effects. I personally think it is God's way of slowing us down. I use that time for silent meditation.

It is recommended that your head go down on the pillow when the sun goes down. While living in a time-change zone, you may actually need to go to bed earlier for enough sleep until sunrise. This can usually be accomplished using an eye cover.

These recommendations may sound time-consuming; however, it is almost impossible to find a person who cannot use this amount of time in place of television or some other nonessential activity or entertainment. Remember investing a little time in this plan will make all your activity healthier, more enjoyable, and more efficient.

My major is business administration. I remember an office management class which recommended the best use of time. The priority was to do the most difficult task first. After that, everything was downhill.

Time

To master time is built into you. Choose to stop giving in to time. Time waits for no one, but time is not your enemy. Make time your friend. Respect time by removing TV time or whatever consumes your time and replace these times with the recommendations in this book. You will be healthier for it.

You can make time your ally by keeping regular hours and eat and sleep on a regular schedule. Avoid drastic changes in diet and activity. Make a healthy work environment. Reduce distractions. Rest quietly once to twice during the day to let your body retune itself. Take yourself out of a stressful situation sooner rather than later.

Take your time; don't rush. Make decisions when they arise. Don't procrastinate or get distracted. Pay attention to what is directly in front of you. Focus on one thing at a time. Don't multitask. Dividing your attention leads to confusion and weakened focus. Yes, I multitasked for years, and it was mostly exhausting.

Avoid the temptation to plunge into high-risk situations. Stay within your comfort zone. Put your house and finances in order. Become more resilient emotionally. Live as if you have all the time in the world. Once you have conquered the basics listed above, then you can go outside your comfort zone if needed for some good reason (for example, asking people to church or how you can pray for them).

If you have already decided on your plan of attack to be healthier, you may consider the hardest part for you and attacked that first. Then everything is smooth sailing. Please do not forget the detox which can reset your body clock. Becoming more alert and clear-headed may surprise you, but it is normally what happens after cleaning your diet. Medically speaking, the body precisely calibrates the correct biochemical balance for a full day's activity when you feed it only the proper nutrients.

Addictions

Fifty million Americans are addicted to tobacco products. Two hundred forty million people around the world are dependent on alcohol, with fifty-five million in America caught driving under the influence of alcohol. Drug overdose deaths have tripled since 1990. Many searches on the Internet proved difficult to get the millions who are addicted to drugs, addicted to prescriptions (also drugs), and the approximate number on drugs of some kind. It is staggering.

All these addictions and any other harmful addiction is a sign of a serious loss of balance. Loss of balance can be described as a distortion of intelligence. Do not waste your time attacking definitions of addiction and how it applies to the physical body or brain. Focus on the hope you have to overcome the addiction. Yes, following the plan in this book to cleanse your body and brain is helpful, but also many will need additional help. That help may come from meditation or prayer.

Many addictions which are a habit are rooted in memory. Many addicts will forgo their habit automatically when offered a greater source of satisfaction. It is hard to believe now; but meditation, especially on God and what he wants for your life, renews your nervous system's memory. This creates a balance, eventually a perfect balance. Meditate or pray as often as you can every day. It will allow your mind to focus on the greater satisfaction. Regular meditation or prayer provides stability. Find your greater satisfaction that is not harmful.

Studies have shown that the longer you practice meditation or prayer, the less dependent one is on addiction. This is usually not a fast fix. Some drug addicts may take as long as one to two years. It sure beats the alternative. Statistical studies tend to be about people we do not know. Therefore, I can personally tell you, from observing people over half a century, that many have been able to quit their addiction when they realized the greater satisfaction was living for God. You can extrapolate the results from the many situations where people are successful.

They made a choice to choose God. Many attribute this to saving their life. This ability exists in every one of us. Whether you reach this point through meditation, prayer, or some other decision, you realize you have accepted that decision. Remember no decision is a decision.

The addiction to alcohol or drugs often has symptoms that are practically indistinguishable from mental illness. This is where we see the correlation between memory being unbalanced and quantum healing. God still performs miracles; however, most people are not cured by miracles. At the quantum level, we are all master builders. It is necessary only to follow the guiding intelligence of our nature, and the vast complexity of the body will run as perfectly as the seasons.

Even if we did not have a duty to our family, to be healthy to support our family, we owe it to God to be healthy. You are entitled to perfect health, and God wants you to be healthy. God has given us the perfect balance we need. We just need to recognize it and act upon it.

This whole-body quantum healing is the cutting edge of physics for our time. If you choose to be courageous on this journey of life, you will not see yourself being confined by boundaries. You realize now the self-knowledge you have can give you the ultimate freedom and the life God intended for you. God gives you wisdom and also sends people to help you. If you have prayed for an answer, receive this book as that answer. Follow the plan in this book, followed with prayer and meditation. Be gentle in your approach.

Associate and spend time with other believers, especially healthy, normal people with common sense. People with common sense should not tell you it does not matter what you eat. Or it does not matter how much sleep you get or if you exercise or not or if you stay clean or if you should truly love God the way the Bible says. Do what you need to stay focused on God and what he wants for you. He wants you to be healthy and happy. He also wants you to eat good, healthy food, get enough sleep, and exercise.

Love God

There's a movie by Kendrick Brothers *Facing the Giants*. It points to what's most important in life, which is God. The best way to validate your existence is to accept God by accepting his son, Jesus Christ. This is the most important thing in life that you can do. If you want to serve God properly with your whole life and face the giants in your life, you should be healthy. This book offers you the opportunity to do that.

I had (and have) the absolute pleasure of learning from sermons preached by evangelists, ministers, preachers, pastors, and other religious leaders during my lifetime. Rhys Stenner is the senior pastor at New Hope Church and brings a fresh message each time, where we are fed and equipped so we can live the life God has called us to live. Tim Woodruff is a minister who preaches and teaches classes about equipping believers to be disciples and light to the world. He inspires courage and perseverance. Dan Cathy is an instrument of God. Once he preached about Jesus washing feet and brought brushes for us to clean a stranger's feet (shoes). This hands-on act humbled us to the point that we will never forget that service of love. Dr. Talmadge French and his two sons, Ryan and Nathan, deliver powerful sermons focusing on Jesus and how to live the daily life in Christ. This wealth of knowledge has given me wisdom to know what is the most important thing in life you can do, salvation, and how to pray.

God is all the wonderful things Christians say he is. He is also a God who expects you to do your part. Do you know how many times in the Bible the word *if* appears? You might be surprised to learn that most, if not all, of God's blessings flow to you after the *if.* If you seek him, you will find him, if you confess with your mouth that he is Lord.

The best way to glorify God, know God, serve God, is to do what he asks of you, to accept his son, Jesus, as the only way to him. Yes, you guessed it, he also wants you to treat your body as a temple in which his Holy Spirit can work. Do not defile his temple, your body, by feeding it garbage. Yes, it is in the Bible; your body is a temple for him. Make a decision today to live for him, accept his son, Jesus, and treat your body like a temple. I see it as one complete package.

I know many people who either do not believe in God, do not believe he exists, or at least will tell you that, or exhibit no relationship to God, Jesus, or the Holy Spirit. Some of these people are very healthy and appear to be happy; and that is because they eat right, get enough sleep, and exercise. I know many Christians, people who genuinely love God, live for God, and do all of the right things, but are unhealthy. It is because they do not eat right, get enough sleep, and exercise. I know that God can perform miracles, but he gives us free will to choose. We are expected by God to make the right decisions, including what we eat. Can God heal you if you are sick? Absolutely. However, my experience in life is that the majority of the time, he does not heal the person.

I hear people say that God did heal the person. It was just on the other side, after the person died and went to heaven. I have no argument with that statement. My point is that you do not get to continue to live in this life being healthy and happy absent good choices, starting with what you decide to eat.

Good things and bad things happen to good people. Good things and bad things happen to bad people. These statements are now in a religious movie. I was saying this before the movie and added, "But you have one choice. Do you go through the good things and bad things (life) with God or without God?"

If you do not have a couple of favorite scriptures from the Bible, find them. Learn them, memorize them, and you will be able to draw strength from them at any moment. Most people know John 3:16, and that is very important. I love Romans 12:1–2 because it tells you exactly how to do God's will.

For those who doubt the evidence in the Bible, I recommend the many interpretive books, CDs, and DVDs by evangelist Perry Stone. The first prophecy I heard him reveal was why David selected five stones to fight Goliath. The first one took down Goliath and four remained. Why? It was a prophecy, as you read later in 2 Samuel where Goliath's four relatives came later to kill David.

Those of you who doubt that there is a God, I recommend *The Case for Christ* by Lee Strobel. He was an atheist who went on a journey to prove his position. The historian Josephus also has good insights into the proof for Christ. Deepak Chopra, who knows way more about health than most, opines that your body is the junction between the visible and the invisible worlds.

Regardless of belief in religion, there is an understanding I have based on my upbringing. We are spiritual beings, and our body connects our physical self and mind to God through our soul and spirit. The last thing I heard my Uncle Bob say before he left this world was that God wants his children to be happy. I will add healthy and happy. Absolutely God can do good from something bad. He also gives you a brain so you can choose to make right decisions. Make godly decisions, so he can bless you abundantly, more than you can ask or imagine.

Pray the Jabez prayer. It asks God to bless you. This is not selfish. God loves you!

There are many books with information about enlightenment. My book focuses on the practical hands-on application. Believe in God, trust God, but do your part he wants you to do. You will receive enlightenment when you believe in God and follow his direction as outlined in his word, the Bible. Go get the knowledge. I like the line by Jimmy Stewart playing George Bailey in *It's a Wonderful Life*. He said he wanted to see what they know. He was talking about traveling abroad and then college to gain all the knowledge he could.

This book contains the nuggets of gold from hundreds of health books and religious interpretive books. It also removes the superfluous material that might hinder you getting a grasp of what's important. God's Word tells us to ask and you will receive. Can it be that simple? Absolutely.

Believe you can change. Decide to make that change. If you truly love yourself the way God loves you, you will make that change to be a healthier, happier person.

This book does not discuss karma. That is for other authors. The focus here is on free will given to us by the God of the universe, the one and only true God, the father of Jesus. Determine to follow him and receive what he wants for your life. That is undoubtedly to be healthy and happy.

We have heard our entire lives to use words of love, encouragement, and positive thoughts. When a person hears these words, it makes a change in their brain. We know we can choose how we respond to any comment, but your response is so much easier when you are responding to positive words.

Joy

Joy can help you lower your stress, lower your risk of heart attack, improve your blood pressure, boost your immune system, help you focus, improve your memory, cause you to want to serve others, make you more grateful and content, help you lose weight, and give you a better outlook on life.

God wants you to have joy.

> If you keep my commandments, you will abide in my love [really cool]...that my joy may be in you, and that your joy may be full. (John 15:10–12)

> In your presence, there is fullness of joy. (Psalm 16:11)

May he grant you your heart's desire and fulfil all your plans! May we shout for joy over your salvation. (Psalm 20:4–5).

Pray about your heart's desires because it can mean he gives you "his desires" as "your heart's desires" because he always wants what's best for you.

Love and Marriage

Experimenters at Harvard have shown the immediate effect of love on the body. Subjects sat in a room to watch a film of Mother Theresa and her work with abandoned children in Calcutta. As the viewers watched the deeply moving images, their breathing rate and blood chemistry changed, revealing greater calm and less stress. These responses are controlled by the brain.

If even a brief exposure to higher love creates a new brain response, what about the effects of love in the long run? Older couples who enjoy a good marriage have been studied, and they report that they love each other more after thirty or forty years than when they first fell in love. But they also report that it's a different kind of love, not the overwhelming infatuation that poets compare to madness but a steadier, more constant, deeper love. You may not feel that wild passionate love like you did when you first met your spouse, but as the years progress, you can have a steadier, more constant, deeper love.

Healthy energy is flowing, flexible, dynamic, balanced, and associated with positive feelings. Unhealthy energy is stuck, frozen, rigid, brittle, hard, out of balance, and associated with negative emotions. Keep your energy healthy by eating right, getting enough sleep and exercising so you can achieve the balance you need.

Equally Yoked

Since what the author desires is to give you a complete package, I have included certain information about your partner that will reduce your stress. Make no mistake about it; the best advice is in the Bible. "Be ye equally yoked." That means before you decide to make a person your permanent partner, make sure you are yoked equally in spirit. This is not any spirit. It is the Holy Spirit from God. Make sure your potential partner, hopefully even before you date, has the same moral values. A great book describing this is *Boundaries in Dating* by John Townsend and Henry Cloud.

My takeaway from this book is that you should not be even dating a person that you do not believe will be your spouse. While you might be seeking a little variety in your dating, you could be with that person you know is not right while God was orchestrating the right one for you. You may miss that opportunity for the one God wants for you.

I was married before and went for all the things I wanted. My wife I have is the one God chose for me. That happened because I totally surrendered to God and sought his will according to Romans 12:1–2. No one is perfect, but I believe you will have a much better chance if you allow God to be involved in your selection process.

I hear a spouse say that the other spouse completes them. This sounds good. I may have even said it myself. However, you need to be whole and complete by yourself. This is total awareness, and you are enough. Your spouse can be the love of your life and compliment you, but no one except you should complete you. Wholeness thinking can set you free. Wholeness is yours if you want it.

Do not confuse this thinking with accepting Jesus as your savior. Of course, he removes your sin and makes you whole spiritually. I have experienced God and know that he is real. The wholeness of mind to which I refer is your simple decision to use the wisdom God gave you to decide to become healthy and happy.

Financial

Since the number one reason for marital discourse is finances, I should address it for this book.

Obviously, you should try not to quit a job until you have another job. Do not spend more than you make. Pay God his tithe. You cannot outgive God. Allocate some portion of your income even small to savings.

Some people even succumb to stress in the opposite direction. They are making enough income but save too much. A retirement program is good, but don't put so much in the retirement account that you are living close to poverty. Although we all want to be healthy, which has a good side effect of living longer, we are not guaranteed tomorrow. Some portion of your income should go for fun like entertainment. Some portion of your retirement may be enjoyed now instead of waiting for some future age.

My spouse and I paid tithes when we were actually spending more than our income for years. We were blessed and now enjoy life to the fullest while having savings and a good inheritance for our children. The more we give to churches, ministries, missions, and God's people, the more we are blessed. We do not do it for that reason. I think that may be why we are so blessed.

King Solomon, David's son, recorded in the Bible, asked God for wisdom. God gave him wisdom and riches. When you ask God for wisdom, do not expect the riches, but perhaps you will be surprised. Think outside the box, be creative, but follow your handbook, the Bible. The joy, fun, and even excitement is worth more than money in the bank. When you reach this point to have this kind of peace, it helps you be healthy.

Destiny or Fate

A person once told me that if he were supposed to be in church, it would happen. This is baloney, as people say in the south. Baloney is full of junk. You must think about it, plan it, set the clock the night before, and go to bed on time. God can do anything, but he gives us the choice and the freedom; so when we choose him, it is delightful.

We must be intentional about serving God. We must also be intentional about our health. Think about it, plan it, make notes, set dates or deadlines, and you can make it happen when you decide to do so. Find a peace about what you want to do. Our daughter Fawn always loves everybody and never criticizes. This approach of loving others can help you find your destiny.

Research on Willpower

Roy Baumeister and John Tierney wrote *Willpower: Rediscovering the Greatest Human Strength.* Ultimately, self-control lets you relax because it removes stress and enables you to conserve willpower for the important challenges. Learning to get willpower and apply it in your daily life can make your life more productive, fulfilling, easier, and happier. Use your self-control to form a daily habit, and you'll produce more with less effort in the long run.

Self-control is not selfish. Willpower enables us to get along with others and override impulses that are based on personal short-term interest. Temporary interests can be controlling. Self-control will be most effective if you take good basic care of your body, starting with diet and sleep.

Kelly McGonigal wrote *The Willpower Instinct: How Self-Control Works, What Matters, and What You Can Do to Get More of It.* Neuroscientist have discovered that when you ask the brain to meditate, it gets better not just at meditating but at a wide range of self-control skills, including attention, focus, stress management, impulse control, and self-awareness. Your body was born to resist cheesecake (or your favorite dessert). Self-control is a matter of physiology, not just psychology. The good news is that you can learn to shift your physiology into the state when you need your willpower the most. You can also train the body's capacity to stay in this state so that when temptation strikes, your instinctive response is one of self-control.

Many factors influence your real power reserve, from what you eat (plant-based and unprocessed foods help; junk food does not) to where you live (poor air quality decreases heart rate variability). Anything that puts a stress on your mind or body can interfere with the physiology of self-control. Exercise is the closest thing to a wonder drug that self-control scientists have discovered.

Desire is the brain's strategy for action. It can be both a threat to self-control and a source of willpower. When dopamine points us to temptation, we must distinguish wanting from happiness. Progress can be motivating and even inspire future self-control but only if you view your actions as evidence that you are committed to your goal. In other words, you need to look at what you have done and conclude that you must really care about your goal so much so that you want to do even more to reach it. What matters is where we let it point us and whether we have the wisdom to know when to follow.

The most effective stress-relief strategies are exercising or playing sports, praying or attending a religious service, reading, listening to music, spending time with friends or family, getting a massage, going outside for a walk, meditating or doing yoga, and spending time with a creative hobby. The least effective strategies are gambling, shopping, smoking, drinking, eating, playing video games, surfing the Internet, and watching TV or movies for more than two hours.

Resolve to feel good. Remember that the future self who receives the consequences of our present self's actions is indeed still us and will very much appreciate the effort. Our human nature includes both the self that wants immediate gratification and the self with a higher purpose. We are born to be tempted and born to resist.

With willpower, you can train your mind and your body. We can recognize our natural capacity for self-control, even if we sometimes struggle to use it. People who have the greatest self-control aren't waging war. They have learned to accept and integrate these competing selves.

If there is a secret for greater self-control, it points to one thing: the power of paying attention. It's training the mind to recognize when you're making a choice rather than running on autopilot. It's remembering what you really want and knowing what really makes you feel better. Self-awareness is the one you can always count on to help you do what is difficult and what matters most. With willpower, you also fully recognize living for God is the best, and you have not missed anything important.

By example, psychoanalysis has largely faded from the scene, replaced by drug therapies for mental disorders. There is no pill for happiness in the medicine cabinet. However, pain and suffering are not essential. Remember willpower is the function of blood sugar. You must clean your diet, eat right, which means only healthy foods, and your blood sugar will reach the point of allowing you to have amazing willpower, not just willpower for food but willpower for everything in your life. It sounds too good to be true, but this time it is true. You will never go wrong by following simple advice I think we all learned in the third grade.

Silence

I love oldies music and play that music in my car. However, there are times when I ride in silence. It is soothing to my inner self.

When visiting the restroom, do not get in a hurry. This is an opportunity to have at least a couple minutes of meditation to rejuvenate. Sit while returning water even if you are a male. Relax every muscle in your body. It causes less stress, and the bathroom will be cleaner.

If you can do stretching in complete silence, you can meditate or pray, whichever is more soothing for you. You will achieve more peace in your soul. When you use the restroom, do so in silence, uninterrupted. These times during the day should be used for meditation and relaxing. You are in charge of your life.

I believe most people talk to themselves or communicate with themselves throughout the day. Some actually do this audibly. They seem to get a benefit from this communication. Know that this may be normal for them. I usually ask, "Who is winning." Tell yourself you will do this challenge to be silent and succeed.

Open Mind

I learned from a good friend Pastor Dr. John P. Avant that it is good to keep an open mind. Years ago, a movie was released with Tom Hanks called *The Da Vinci Code*. Many religious people were commenting that Christians should not see the movie. However, John said he went to see it because he wanted to know and have the information available to intelligently talk to other people about Jesus and the truths in the Bible. That sounded well-reasoned, and I saw the movie. I was not only entertained but given information I did not know, so I can intelligently talk about different views.

Pastor John Avant taught me many things, especially how to confidently ask someone, even a stranger, how I can pray for them. The first time I did this at a restaurant, the server said, "Yes, my daughter has cancer." She put out her hands to pray with my wife and I then. People are hurting and want someone to care. I did it for the right reasons because I was genuinely concerned. It had a mutual benefit though; I then realized I could be a mouth or hands for God to a complete stranger. It reduces stress when you help someone.

Pray to have an open mind and an open heart to receive what God has for you. I believe he wants you to be healthy and happy.

Choices

Your choices each played a part in the body you created (over the years). Every time you exercise, you alter your skeleton and muscles. Every bite of food you eat alters your daily metabolism, electrolyte balance, and proportion of fat to muscle.

Your body is alive with unknown abilities, but it looks to you for direction. Mental activity alone can alter the brain. You need to trust your body's cues when eliminating food. I have eliminated a particular food more than once to verify the results. Congratulate yourself for being willing to change. Appreciate your body for its honesty. Remain centered, which is a state of calm and stability. Tell your mind that this will work and you can do it. When your diet becomes cleaner, you will be clear thinking, which brings more clarity to what's important in life.

Expect the best. Some people may need to surrender themselves to this thought. That's okay, remember, whatever it takes to get to healthy living and feeling good every day.

Prayer and Chain and Ring

Your mental health will be helped greatly if you seek to help other people. This can be done so easily. Asking them how you can pray will give you specifics upon which you can pray. Always remember you can put feet and hands to those prayers.

Another way to help people is using the chain and ring. My wife and I have been all around the world sharing this with others. It is simply a two-foot thin chain like you would have for a dog tag around a service person's neck joined with a clip and a two-inch metal ring. The story is that the chain is big (around) like God. The ring is small like us. And if you have faith, he will not let you fall, probably more appropriately is to say "when you fall, he will catch you." There is a video online that shows how to do this. Once the person repeats the story to me, I give it to them, always no charge.

We use it as a ministry tool on mission trips and on our regular vacations around the world. It brings a lot of joy to many, especially children.

Forgiveness

Your mental attitude is a huge factor in your health. If there is any unforgiveness in your life, get rid of it. All experts will tell you that unforgiveness or bitterness will hurt you more than the other person.

There are many books written on how to move forward after a harmful or hurtful event. Suffice it to say that you need to do whatever you need to do, legally, to move forward without the unforgiveness or bitterness. My recommendation from reading these materials is to make a definitive choice you will not harbor any unforgiveness or bitterness! To accomplish this, focus on all the good information in this book to accept God, trust God, and move forward by making yourself healthy, your body and your mind.

Be careful about using any drugs, prescription or not. Google anything you are taking to read the side effects. Often the side effects are more dangerous than the reason you're taking the drug. I give no medical advice in this book but unequivocally will tell you that I know many people who have changed their diet and eliminated all drugs, including over-the-counter medications. If there is a drug that absolutely cannot be avoided, everything in this book should help you minimize any side effects.

Once your brain is unaffected by drugs, you have a better chance of moving forward optimistically. You then can more easily resolve any unforgiveness or bitterness. When you truly surrender to God, you will love him the way you should, you will accept his beliefs as your beliefs, and you will live in freedom. There's a scripture in the Bible that says forsake yourselves not to assemble together. This means believers should be in the corporate body like the church so all members can work together. If everyone had the attitude that I can just watch church on television and there were no churches, how many people do you think would accept Jesus as their savior? Not many I can tell you.

If we decided not to attend church regularly, we would not be properly equipped for the ministry. We would miss unity, become stagnant and isolated, become more easily deceived by false teachings. We would neglect using our gifts to their fullest and miss the opportunities to be encouraged and experience true love. Scripture shows that it is God's design for you to be the church and in church with other believers.

Be intentional, especially when saying that you love God. He calls us to accept him but also to tell others. If you are a believer, how did you become a believer? I don't think it was sitting outside looking at the trees. Of course, anything is possible with God, so don't look for an exception to avoid what God commands us to do.

Our minister of prayer Hugh Kirby says that the Bible is God's love letters to us. These commands should be recognized for what they are, which is love to protect us and keep us truly free. He also reminds us to do popcorn prayers, which are done when the need arises.

I have heard, "God said it, I believe it, and that settles it." That's not entirely accurate. "God said it, and that settles it." It doesn't matter whether you believe it. However, God gives you a choice to accept him. It would be wise to do that regardless of circumstances.

Beyond Control

Nothing is impossible with God. Very little is out of your control. The human will to survive is so strong. Use that will to get healthy. If you decide to do so, it will happen.

According to God in the Bible, heaven will be more awe-striking than when we experienced the movie *The Passion of the Christ*. Everyone who left the movie could not speak. We are God's children. Dwell on that.

Major Truths

Major truths in life are irrefutable. One is that if you eat a clean healthy diet, you will be healthier. If you are healthier, you will sleep better. If you sleep better, you'll feel like exercising (more). If you wash your hands, especially now, before touching your face, and keep clean, you will be healthier. If you love God by following his manual for life, the Bible, you will be healthier, especially your mental health will be better.

Pray to God and ask him to reveal the major truths for your life. Jesus is the Truth according to the Bible.

Soul

It is easy to connect with your soul. Jesus said, "Ask and you shall receive." When you sincerely ask and believe, you can receive it. Your soul, Jesus, and salvation are the keys. They connect you to God who is the creator of the universe.

Your healthy body brings clarity, which allows you to understand the major truths in life. Read your Bible when you are sick, and you may be desperate. You should read it at all times. Read your Bible when you are healthy, and you will understand more.

Look at the need the soul fulfills. Functioning as your spiritual body, the soul generates and organizes the energy of love and compassion and the awareness of truth, creativity, and intelligence. That way, it fulfills the needs that are just as basic as the need of the physical body for food and oxygen.

The human potential can reach amazing heights, especially when plugged in to God. Loving God means knowing God and his Word. A sincere desire to know God will lead you to read, study, and apply his Word in your life daily.

First and foremost is accepting his son, Jesus, as your savior. After that, you are to tell others. If you received a fantastic Christmas present, you most likely will tell others. Salvation is more than one million times better than the best Christmas present. Loving God like this gives you a freedom and wisdom that can allow you to make the right choices. Make godly choices to treat your body like a temple. It is a temple for God.

Living like this gives you an enormous advantage over nonbelievers. Pray for them, but seize your destiny. Embrace the new. Use creativity, and consider moving outside your comfort zone (in this situation). You will find the most inspiring and pleasurable moments in your life.

Although we know God wants what's best for us, sometimes we try to be God. Realize that he is God, and he can do anything he wants. The Bible is our instruction manual. If you do not have God living through the Holy Spirit in you, finding God is easier than trying to be God.

Your body thrives on sunlight. Every bite of food represents trapped sunlight that your body releases into chemical and electrical energy. Your cells have no future except through light. Your soul has no future except through Jesus. It is interesting that our physical body relies on *sun*, and our spiritual body relies on *Son*.

Our choices are endless, but focus on love for God first. Put God's kingdom first. Knowing, being creative, spontaneous, dynamic, playful, and ever expanding are the other choices, which help us live the life we were intended to live.

Give peace where you can. I remember inviting a pastor to lunch. I have been doing this for many years over my lifetime and really enjoy taking pastors to lunch. This particular time, my wife and I met the pastor in the restaurant at the assigned time, and there was an air of uncertainty. We believed that he thought we had invited him to lunch to make a complaint. I have never complained when inviting a pastor to lunch. We merely wanted to enjoy his company. Within the first few minutes, I told him that we had no agenda and just wanted to enjoy talking to him during lunch. You could immediately see the change in his countenance. His face was relaxed, and we had a very enjoyable time.

People may be reluctant to accept your request to meet for lunch even if it is arranged to be dutch, each pay his own. I have found over my lifetime that many pleasant and enjoyable minutes can be realized while having a meal together. Yes, it is good to conduct business during a meal, but sometimes just enjoying the person is enough.

Either you believe the Bible, or you don't. God can handle anything. Give your prayers to God without claw marks.

Awareness

You learned everything you need to know in the third grade. Eat right, get enough sleep, exercise, wash your hands, and love God. We know the priority is loving God first. However, this order was mentioned because if you don't eat right, get enough sleep, and exercise, you will not be able to or feel like loving God the way you should (repeated for emphasis). It is important to get your mind right before you try to get your body right.

What is the most important thing in life? That can be debated for days; however, I maintain that salvation through God our Creator is the priority. Therefore, understand who God is. Some people might say the most important thing in life is God, glorifying God, or knowing God. None of these will get you to the ultimate priority unless you have salvation. Without salvation, none of this life means anything.

If you go through life, die, and that is the end of it, what is the real purpose? Of course, you can rationalize that during your life you helped people, made a difference, or achieved certain goals. These are wonderful things, but salvation for you and others means eternal life. If you are a believer or decide to be a believer, you will understand that the big picture is that we are only on earth for a very short period of time (a speck in eternity). When teaching children in Sunday school, I will draw a dot on the board and a long line after the dot going off the end of the board. The dot represents all of your life on earth and the line represents eternity with God. God only asks us to live for him for this speck in time, and he offers forever with him in heaven. What kind of deal is that? Please tell me that you understand this truth.

If you read and understand the Bible, you will know that God is real. God is alive, not just in nature but in a way where his spirit can live inside you. There is a song in the movie *God's Not Dead*, "My Gods not dead, he's surely alive, living on the inside, roaring like a lion, God's not dead." This is a good way to understand how God lives in us.

There may seem to be inconsistencies in the Bible. With these interpretive books, you can reconcile those apparent differences. The apparent differences actually give corroboration to the Scriptures. God breathed the words through men who did act as a human filter; so Matthew, Mark, Luke, and John give similar stories but none that are inconsistent with the intent of scripture. Prayer and reading the Bible have helped people understand the truth in the Bible without interpretive books.

The Bible says the Truth is Jesus, the son of God. Without Jesus, there is no salvation. I pray that you understand what the Bible says, that Jesus is the only way to God the Father. Jesus is the only one, of many so-called gods, who is still alive. All the others, including Mohammed, Buddha, etc., are dead. The others do not even claim to still be alive. Over five hundred people saw Jesus after he rose from the dead. The evidence of this is overwhelming when you consider reporting practices and other influencers during that time.

I have been teaching Sunday school for most of my adult life, over a quarter of a century teaching the children. The sixth graders when told, "You learned everything you need to know in the third grade. Eat right, get enough sleep, exercise, wash your hands, and love God," will say, "No sir, we learned that in the first grade." Even schools, along with good parents, have taught our youth what's important in life.

Just in a practical sense, without breaking the boundary of blasphemy, consider two people going through life. The first person believes Jesus is the way, lives his life accepting Jesus and living for Jesus, turning from his sin and seeking to live as a Christian. The second person does not believe in Jesus as the way. He may even live just like a Christian but does not accept Jesus as her savior. If what God told us in the Bible is *not* true, the first person lived a great, fulfilling, rewarding life anyway, the second person also with what appears to be a good life. However, if what God tells us in the Bible *is* true, the first person goes to heaven and lives forever with God in a place we can barely begin to describe as wonderful. The second person clearly does not go to heaven, and he is destined to spend eternity without God in pain and torment. God gives us free will to not be a robot but so we can choose God (or not).

While on the subject, we must entertain the worldwide question of how can a loving God allow so much pain and suffering. You cannot have free will without the choices. God loved us so much that he gave away part of his power and authority to us, as free will. He actually lets us choose to make good choices or bad choices. God tells us in his Word he wants us to choose him. However, he also tells us in his Word that he knows some will not choose him.

It appears simple. You have two choices. You can choose to go through life with God, or you can choose to go through life without God. It may be an oversimplification, but it explains how easy it can be to see the light. The light is Jesus. *Is Genesis History?* (and *Beyond Is Genesis History?*) DVDs and documentary give additional clear proof that the Bible and God are true and real.

Positive Thoughts

Tell yourself positive thoughts every day. You are important. You are smart. You are kind. I believe those things about you as a reader since you chose this book. As you think, you are. When you are healthy, you can have full awareness of self. Then when you speak to another person, your awareness speaks to theirs, and that is enough to create changes in the brain.

It is actually unhealthy to worry about your health. *The Helsinki study* proved this. This book is not intended in any way to make you worry. See what you can use gently and maybe slowly to change your health for the better. As you get healthier, you will decide to perhaps do more, to eat a better diet, to exercise more, to really get the sleep you need.

When you're fully aware, you can center yourself at will. You are familiar with the place of peace and silence inside. You are not divided against yourself nor inner conflicts. You can transcend local disturbances and remain unaffected by them. You see the world from an expanded perspective. And your inner world is organized. This is what it means to rise above cravings.

What is a dream hospital stay? What would be all your favorite things? To have complete rest and sleep from 8:00 p.m. to 6:00 a.m.? To have the right fluids and food upon request? Have a massage and a person exercise your limbs to prevent atrophy? Everything just the way you want so you have complete peace of mind? This describes, with the possible exception of massaging, what I experience each day basically, all while in the comfort of my own home.

Good decisions are always rewarded. Many rewards occur in heaven, but many occur on earth. Our eldest daughter Reba wrote something recently.

> When I tell you that he would be at everything he could for his children and grandchildren, I really mean it. To a soccer game for one, football game for another, visiting grandchildren in a different city, and having dinner with another one in the same day. He has cut his trips short just to be with us children. I remember waking to the smell of breakfast. Every Sunday without fail we would go to church. We wouldn't just go to church, we had to get up and dressed nice and show God that we cared about his day. Little did I know that would end up being the foundation of my love for our Savior. My Daddy has made an effort as he still does to reach out to his [grown] children several times per week. I never had a period where he was absent and I am forever grateful. I try to show him in how I love my children and how I love my Lord, that those things people think are actually what shape who you are. Live your life like you want your children to live theirs. When my Daddy says he is proud of me I remind him that I am him in so many ways.

Intentional

Many times in my life, I have heard people say, "Well, you have to die from something." However, I say, "You shouldn't hasten it." I do not eat right, get enough sleep, and exercise as well as staying clean and being faithful to God to live longer. I do it to feel good every day. I am willing to do what it takes to feel good. Again, feeling good is not overrated. Finding strength and comfort from your spiritual faith has been proven by researchers to show you are seven times more likely to survive a stressful event, especially a major surgery. If you are discounting God, you do it at your own peril. Being in church is usually not enough. Remember the key words are *strength and comfort from your spiritual faith*.

It is important that you feel loved every day. This is where God will never fail you. The Bible can be called a book of love stories. These are stories from God to you. You should feel loved every day. If there is ever any day that you do not feel loved, read your Bible, especially first Corinthians. If you still need help, talk to your pastor, minister, accountability partner, or another strong believer.

Attitude

Regardless of circumstances, you have the ability to choose how you react and feel. Choose to smile and laugh every chance you get. I confess it is not always easy. Make a decision every morning that you will look for opportunities to help others. This will give you an expectation of fulfillment. This should allow you to smile and hopefully laugh many times during the day. Our son Dave is always laughing. Although he had difficulty with choices at one time (like most of us), he pulled through, probably because he always finds humor in everything. He chose to persevere.

If you read the Bible with an attitude for sincerely wanting to know God's will for your life, especially Romans 12:1–2, you can know what it is. Then you will be able to awaken every morning excited and go to sleep every night fulfilled. The Bible is true. Jesus is who he says he is. God is his Father, and Jesus returned to heaven and sent the Holy Spirit to his people on earth. The Holy Spirit is yours if you accept Jesus as your savior.

You have the right to remain silent. This means you can choose to be optimistic and talk about only the good. My mother always said if you cannot say something good, don't say anything. If you need a little help to laugh, try *Octogenarians Say the Darndest Things!* written by David L. Anders, MD, with Rebekah Yates Anders, MD. If you want a hilarious start, sneak ahead, and first read Jeff Foxworthy on page 18, "You might be growing older if…"

Rationalize

Humans can rationalize anything, even murder. So rationalize that you can do this program.

Rules

In order to understand the rules which apply to bring you a healthier lifestyle, remember the basics.

- You learned everything you need to know in the third grade.
- You control your own body with your own choices.
- You are conscious and can make your own choices.
- Everything fits together. Each choice absolutely affects something.
- Organizing your thoughts based on the information in this book will be positive.
- Freedom results from your positive decisions.

A detox and cleaning your diet require a fraction of your time. When you are feeling good every day and looking back on your decisions, you will feel good, very good. My friend and partner Daniel Kalamaro says that after you get your diet clean, where it should be, if you backslide, you notice it more. After a night with ice cream, the next morning when he ran, which is always good and fun, he thought he would die. A little in moderation (so called) can be unhealthy. Although he sweats out the toxins as he calls it, it was not the feel-good to which he is accustomed. It did not kill him, but for me, I just don't eat ice cream. I like feeling good all the time.

However, I, like everybody else, backslide at times. The last time I felt so good for so long I thought I could eat foods that were unhealthy. I started slipping slowly by eating a few chips at the restaurant. Then I was eating a whole bowl of chips. I used more and more salad dressing until I realized the amount of sugar in the salad dressing was adversely affecting me. I became light-headed, which meant I lost some clarity and even stability. I was not hindered in my walking, but when toweling dry after a shower, I was not as steady on one foot. I returned to the healthy foods only and recovered quickly. Our body will heal itself quickly if we give it the right nutrients and avoid the harmful foods. Now I need no salad dressing when I have other toppings like fruit, cottage cheese, hummus, etc.

An interesting footnote is that the bad food consumed took about twelve to fourteen hours to register as sickness. My digestive system may be different than those who do not consume only healthy foods for long periods of time. One time in the past, I consumed unhealthy food. Twelve hours later, it surfaced as head spinning, i.e., vertigo. This lasted twenty-four hours. I think it was curtailed because I flushed continuously with water and only ate fruit smoothie, cooked peas, homemade real grits, and a plain omelet during that twenty-four hours. I think sometimes when people say that they had a twenty-four-hour bug, it could have been just a reaction to what they ate. Importantly, for me, during the twenty-four hours, no prescription or over-the-counter drugs were consumed. I think my body was able to fight and heal without having to deal with drugs also. Drugs rarely, if ever, cure anything.

The following cartoon illustrates the current state of affairs for many Americans.

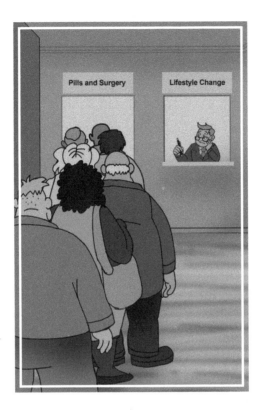

ELSEVIER

Pain

So many people have pain somewhere in their body. Unfortunately, their pain is there often, many times daily. My heart breaks for each person who has pain on a regular basis.

It is well documented that thousands of people have eliminated their pain, even disease and illnesses, by simply changing their diet.

The health books written and published are numerous. If you want proof, you should read them. I have. Or you can read this book and use the nuggets I found that changed my life. Life takes participation. You can participate with ease if you are healthy.

Some people may feel the need to make themselves a promise. Some will make notes. Somebody gets excited and tells their friends.

However, if you do not set a time certain to start this journey, it may never start. When you start, know that you cannot fool yourself. Be honest.

Start with a small lifestyle change, something you can keep and make a habit. Once the habit is formed, you can expand from there. Start by nourishing your body with real whole foods. Commit yourself to the process. Focus on your healthy and happy relationships. Let the Holy Spirit guide you.

If you genuinely want to cooperate with your body, paying it a little attention makes proper diet, sleep, and exercise easy. Your body is going to serve and uphold your interest for a lifetime. The older you get, the more you should be in tune with your body. If your life is to be a great victory, you must win many small battles along the way.

It is unfair and medically false to claim that a depressed patient caused his condition. However, people do contribute to their depression. If you drink too much, engage in toxic relationships, or lack coping skills in times of stress, the result will be depressed brain function.

For many years, when people ask how I am, I respond "marvelous, fantastic, fabulous, living the dream, etc. Ninety percent of my amazing day is done. My outlook and expectations are set. I firmly believe what I am saying." The day follows accordingly.

Do not think because I am a lawyer that is why I am happy. When I was a law-enforcement officer, I was happy. When I was a truck driver, I was happy. The attitude was formed at a very young age and has carried me through life. I promise, if collecting trash tomorrow, I will be happy, seriously. In reality, I am supplying the optimism, expectations, love, the fruit of the spirit, and to the world maybe magic. I believe it, receive it, and act upon it. It is reality.

Filters

As you pursue your journey to optimum health, you may use filters. People can be filters through which you test your ideas or discuss your results. You will bode much better if you use filters of people who are healthy. There are people who never get sick and only go to the doctor for a wellness checkup or physical. Be leery taking advice from someone who is routinely sick. When weighing the advice of others, remember to ultimately intelligently listen to your own body.

Expectations

I have heard people say they attended a particular church for ten years or more and received nothing from the sermons. Wow, that is amazing. In my entire life, I have never sat through one sermon where I did not receive something.

Expectation is powerful. I remember the worst sermon I ever heard, and remember one thing that was very noteworthy. If you expect to get good results by reading this book, you will. That means you will put in practice as many of these suggestions as possible to have a healthy and happy life daily.

Many people are predisposed. I have litigated jury trials where this was exposed in a raw way. Jurors would raise their hands and swear to decide the case only on the facts and law presented in the trial. However, following deliberation and the verdict, the jurors would candidly disclose they did not decide the case that way. All people in the court system, especially litigators and judges, realize that jurors bring with them their life experiences that cannot or will not be disregarded.

This book could be received with cynicism. You are asked to use an open mind to apply what's recommended to see what results are possible for you. If you expect to get good results by reading this book, you will. That means you will put in practice as many of these suggestions as possible to have a healthy and happier life.

Stress

I bragged about having a thirty-three-year litigation career without stress. It is true. However, when I first started the practice of law, I realized that diet was important. So if I had a trial, specifically a jury trial, I would always eat grits, oatmeal, or cream of wheat as a hot cereal that settled my stomach. After five years of practice, I became an arbiter judge in Atlanta; and for twelve years, I decided cases in Fulton Superior Court and Fulton State Court. It provided insight into trying cases. Stress was reduced but mainly by having a good diet.

Truthfully, the only stress I remember is when I broke my leg skydiving and going to the doctor. I have never really been sick during my adult life. My wife makes me go periodically for a physical, although I no longer say I am Superman. The results are always within normal ranges.

In my youth, I ate hamburgers, fries, sodas, pizzas, sugary desserts of all types, and anything I wanted. Of course, I got sick periodically like everybody else. About a quarter of a century ago, I remember getting sick, which was from something I ate. I eliminated that from my stomach and was better quickly. No drugs or pills!

With a high metabolism, I eat four times a day. Of course, I eat a clean diet, so I always feel good. Actually, let's be honest. Ninety-nine percent of the time I feel amazing.

It is important to not take yourself too seriously. Don't sweat the small stuff. You can eliminate almost all the stress by focusing on what is important. Focus on God, good things, helping others, and the things that help you wake excited in the morning and fulfilled in the evening.

Sometimes it is the professor and not the student. Stress seems to be inevitable at times. I had one professor in law school who would ask if we did our homework. He would see a show of hands and tell us to spend the hour studying. He then walked out the door. Many students, including me, had a difficult time learning the topic that quarter. Next quarter, many of us chose another professor, who was ironically a former student of the previous professor, when he was in law school. Every time he would teach, we had an epiphany. We were surprised at how easy it was to learn sitting under his tutelage.

I share that short story with you, so you will know that stress can happen to any of us. However, once again, all the more reason to take care of yourself. If your job requires a lot of thinking, like decision-making, delegating, giving orders, you may want to consider forming your thoughts in the morning. Most people do their best thinking in the morning. Of course, there's an exception to everything.

Don't save good things. Enjoy them now. I know people who have saved things like expensive perfume, china dinnerware, etc. For when? Use those now and enjoy life. You will feel better. Do not wait until you retire to travel, if you like to travel. You may be too tired then.

The icing on the cake for all the medical costs you have saved could be a weekly or biweekly massage. You earned it. Look for a massage school in your area, which often will have more than 50 percent off because the student (masseuse or masseur) is in training. My wife and I have been doing this for years and can tell you they will do what you ask. It can be just as beneficial as the expensive massage. Massage and manipulation can remove poisons from your system.

Yawning can eliminate stress. Not only does it stretch the muscles in your jaw and neck areas, it can relieve any pressure when you are flying. If you travel, make a packing list. It will eliminate all stress of forgetting something. I actually have sections on one page, showing the area of my room or closet. I found that getting everything from the closet at one time was more efficient (same with dresser, bag, etc.). You might be pleasantly surprised. You may also list winter in a subpart, maybe bolded or underlined to show "winter wear."

A river runs fastest on the surface but it's nearly motionless at the bottom. No matter how busy you get, calm yourself inside, your mind, your soul. Every level of the river is the same water and moves toward the same goal. You can do what needs to be done but without stress. Tell yourself there will be no stress in the things you do today.

Forgetful

My whole life I noticed how people at any age can be forgetful. How many of us at almost any age have walked from one room to another and forgot why we went to the other room. Many things we do not believe to be important are sent to that area of our brain that does not allow recall like it does in the other area. The only thing you should fear is fear itself. Fear on almost any level brings stress. If you choose not to be fearful, you will be healthier. Do not confuse fear with safety. We all should strive to be safe and secure at all times. If you really trust God, you can live without fear.

A footnote, since this book involves so much about living healthy, is that if you are becoming more forgetful, remove all sugar, processed, and artificial from your diet. I cannot tell you medically that you will get better, but I certainly did. Although the human body is the same in many ways, we are all different in some ways. It will not hurt to continue cleaning your diet to experiment to see if eliminating certain foods, especially processed sugar, improves your lifestyle. Experimenting absolutely has worked for me my entire life.

Entertainment

Entertainment relieves stress for many people. I found the Kendricks brothers' movies and other Christian movies help relieve stress. They are wholesome and inspiring.

A lot of my buddies are like me. If our car is clean, we feel good. I sincerely mean it is a physical noticeable reaction that occurs in our body. Many hobbies give people the same improved feeling. Find what makes you feel good. Also, if the wheels on a vehicle are clean, that is 90 percent done. For me, preventing any stress regarding cleaning the car means I pay someone else to wash it. We are both happy.

Watching and listening to the daily news is a choice. Most of my life, I have chosen not to watch the news. My spouse always lets me know the one or two important newsworthy items per week. A friend at work may share a newsworthy item.

When adapting to a healthier lifestyle, one consideration may be to eliminate the news. I have always been an optimistic person. I do believe part of this is because I do not flood my brain with the news. Unfortunately, news is mostly bad. Also, if the news starts with a fire, there is no news. This piece of information may save you time.

Most people are not working eighty hours per week and can certainly do what needs to be done to live a healthier life, if they just eliminate television time.

Home Remedies

Why not try home remedies to cure health problems before you see the doctor? Some people suffer from gout. One lady, years ago, during one of her painful experiences from gout, heard that cherry juice would eliminate the pain. Surprisingly, it worked. The pain was completely gone. She drank cherry juice periodically over the next few years and never had any problems.

Fast forward to when the gout returned because she had stopped drinking cherry juice. She went to the doctor with the pain, who prescribed medication, a drug. She had other pain from the side effects from the drug. What happened? Did she forget about the cherry juice? I could not restrain myself from asking why. Her response astounded me. She said, "Well, I just went to the doctor, and he gave me a pill." I think too many people have the mindset that it is easier to go get a pill. It is certainly not healthier.

Today, there is no excuse for not following the EAGLE plan; so you are not required to visit a doctor, sit in the waiting room for who knows how long, pay too much money, and get a drug, which almost always has bad side effects. Ask God to help you, believe that he will, expect a miracle if you will, and move toward first considering a home remedy.

If you have itching, joint pain, or excessive coughing, stop consuming bread and flour. Most people are amazed at the results, with many having complete elimination of the problem. When using a small amount of shampoo, if your scalp still itches, eliminate all flour and bread. This many times will cure the itch. If it is like cradle cap and you have eliminated all the unhealthy foods, you may have another problem. However, it does not hurt to try eliminating foods before spending time and money at the doctor's office.

If you ever have any shoulder pain, try changing sides of the bed first. We tend to rotate during the night toward a particular side. When changing sides, often we will reverse and turn on the other shoulder. This has actually solved the problem for me when I was young, lifting tremendous weights. If it does not solve the problem for you, seek a doctor. Consider muscle stripping before drugs, injections, and surgery. Of course, clean your diet, and do everything you can in your power to avoid drugs, injections, and surgery. When lying on your back—stretching, exercising, or sleeping—and you're feeling nauseous, raise your head until the nausea goes away, usually with a pillow.

In your journey of life, you'll be constantly adapting. Your body changes with the weather, sensing rain or growing calm with the changing of the seasons. Our bodies should intuitively and automatically flow with these changes as long as we do not interfere. The biggest interference often is our diet. In the winter, drink warm or hot water. This may be done with lemon, lime, orange, etc. The body wants and needs the warmth. Warm cooked vegetables are good. In the summer, drink room temperature water and only occasionally with ice as a treat. Your digestive system always works better with room temperature liquids. Eat fresh produce all times of the year, preferably grown locally. If you think about the season, it should be common sense adjusting your eating habits. The seasonal routine should be just another way to encourage your body's own natural instincts to emerge.

In my police career, as a first responder, I saw many people put on a stretcher. So many would scream and beg for their head to be raised. I requested the paramedics to please raise their head. These potential patients may have had more knowledge of their individual situation. Some did not make it when their head was not raised. All the ones I witnessed who had their head raised survived. Even the patients in shock who needed their legs raised still had their head raised and survived. Just my observation during those fifteen years.

A family member should always be with any person who is receiving any form of treatment, if possible.

If you look closely at your own life, you will realize that you are sending signals to your body that repeat the same old beliefs. Accept this plan as a new positive change. It's never too late to begin creating the body we want. You can add many years to your life by deciding to quit smoking, quit tobacco, quit alcohol, and stop drugs. To start, some may want to stop these at least on a regular basis. You can add more years by losing excess weight or eating good food or exercising regularly. These are all very good, but you also need to change your thinking. See yourself as successful in each and every step. Do not entertain the thought of defeat. Don't forget the detox to help you.

This new thinking can be obtained by using the plan in this book. Do it in the order recommended: eating right, getting enough sleep, and exercising. It is really simple. The eating right can go in many different directions, but once you know your body type and follow the diet that matches it, you are on the right track. This will allow for proper digestion and assimilation. It will also allow for the correct elimination which purifies your body. This all must be done daily.

Slow urination may be helped with posture while sitting on the toilet. Most people lean forward and slouch which is acceptable, but also during the same episode, try sitting erect. Often this will allow additional flow. Even leaning to the left can allow additional flow. People are different. Any improvement is better than the risk involved in surgery. Do not put yourself on a time limit going to the restroom. There is nothing wrong with a male taking as long as a female. Of course, these days, so many people look at their phone and stay longer anyway. Slow urination beats surgery any day and gives you additional time to relax and meditate.

In the '50s and before, people would sit on their porch and talk. This was so relaxing. If you have too much stress in your life, you may want to consider reverting to old times. Avoid all electronics and just talk to a friend or family member in person. I see people periodically now get off social media for some length of time. This is good to destress. Most phones now will periodically show you how much time you average on the phone per day. You may be shocked. Why not try easy at-home remedies which may help solve your problem or even completely eliminate your illness. You have the rest of your life to try these at no cost.

The Edgar Cayce Handbook for Health Through Drugless Therapy by Dr. Harold Reilley goes so far as to say if a person eats one almond each day, you will never have accumulations of tumors. If he eats two to three almonds each day, he need not fear cancer. This seems far reaching, especially if you do not have a clean healthy diet. This could be based on the theory that if a person is conscientious enough to do this, that person would probably be eating right to start.

The almond carries more phosphorus and iron and a combination easily simulated than any other nut. However, almonds can be very hard on your teeth, so you may want to consider other nuts like walnuts. Most nuts are good but not peanuts. Some have included cashews with peanuts as nuts not to eat, at least on a regular basis. I eat a small handful of nuts every day as part of my clean diet but rotate the different kinds of nuts to give me a variety. Chew the nuts to a paste before swallowing. I knew people who ate a jar of peanuts at a time and died from cancer. Too many nuts may get caught in your colon. If not removed, they can cause diverticulosis, then diverticulitis, and then develop into colon cancer. Diverticulosis occurs when small bulging pouches (diverticula) develop in your digestive tract. When one or more of these pouches become inflamed or infected, the condition is called diverticulitis. To be extra careful with your colon, I recommend not eating popcorn, corn, seeds unless they are ground, and no nuts unless you chew them to a paste before swallowing.

The study of four hundred cancer cases that went into spontaneous remission revealed cures that had little in common. Some people drank grape juice or swallowed massive doses of vitamin C. Others prayed, took herbal remedies, or simply cheered themselves into a better state of thinking. These very diverse patients did have one thing in common though. At a certain point in their disease, they knew, with complete certainty, that they were going to get better, as if the disease were merely a mirage. The patient suddenly passed beyond the space of fear and despair, and all sickness was nonexistent. They entered the place called perfect health.

I find this information incomplete. It appears that there may have been a common thread not mentioned in this study like a good clean diet. This information is presented for those who may gain strength from the positive thinking offered. I do believe in perfect health. No matter how much you tell yourself you will be healthy; however, if you are consuming poison, you will die. The mental strength is amazing, but you should accompany that with the EAGLE. How much poison should be included in your moderation approach? None! How much of the bad foods and substances should be included in your moderation approach? None!

I, like some others, ended with a pencil stab mark in my hand following elementary school. It was well below the surface of the skin so it was there my entire life. Following my detox and cleaning my diet, one day, I realized it was gone. I cannot explain exactly how, but it was there for fifty years until I changed my diet.

Acid reflux, when you are sleeping, can often be cured by drinking sixteen ounces of water. If this does not work, raise your head. If pillows make too much of an arch to raise your head, raise your mattress under your head or raise the headboard. Headboard can be raised by using blocks of wood one to two inches thick. Often raising the headboard or top of your bed and pillows will suffice.

The so-called secret to health is really simple:

Brain
> As you age, certain parts shrink, blood flow may decrease, and inflammation may increase.
> How to help? Exercise, leafy greens, fatty fish, nuts, B vitamins, and water.

Ears
> As you age, your balance may falter, and hearing loss may occur.
> How to help? Foods rich in magnesium, zinc and potassium, and water.

Lungs

As you age, your diaphragm can weaken, ribs can thin, and lung capacity can reduce.

How to help? Salmon, seeds, preferably ground, cruciferous vegetables, vitamin A, and water

Eyes

As you age, difficulty to focus and differentiate color increases, you may require more light, be more sensitive to glare, and tear production decreases.

How to help? Fatty fish, leafy greens, nuts, omega-3, eggs, vitamin A, C, and E, and water.

Liver

As you age, volume and blood flow decreases, cholesterol volume expands, and regeneration decreases.

How to help? Nuts, fatty fish, berries, and water.

Heart

As you age, arteries can stiffen, plaque can build, heart rate can become irregular, blood pressure can rise.

How to help? Olive oil, avocados, broccoli, vitamins A, E, and K, and water.

Joints

As you age, joints become less flexible and stiffen, and fluid and cartilage may decrease.

How to help? Onions, garlic, walnuts, turmeric, vitamin D, eliminate bread and flour products, and drink water

Kidneys

As you age, tissue and ability to filter blood decreases, and blood vessels harden.

How to help? Berries, fatty fish, spinach, sweet potatoes, B vitamins, and water.

Skin

As you age, outer layer becomes thin, elasticity reduces, blood vessels weaken, and sweat glands produce less.
How to help? Healthy fats, walnuts, vitamins A, B3, and water.

Stomach

As you age, levels of mucus acids and enzymes decrease.
How to help? Olive oil, some resistant starches, cruciferous vegetables, artichokes, mushrooms, vitamin D3, and water.

Muscles

As you age, mass strength and endurance decline.
How to help? Low-fat proteins, leafy greens, omega-3, eggs, nuts, vitamin D, and water.

Bones

As you age, mass and density decline, mineral and calcium loss, spine shortens.
How to help? Greens, sweet potatoes, sardines, calcium, vitamins D, K, and water.

Blood (Mosquitoes prefer type O. I should've known that."

As you age, blood volume decreases, slower response to stress and illness, and reduced infection response.
How to help? Dark greens, lean meats, pomegranates, fatty fish, vitamin C, K, and water.
Notice any consistency? Eat fresh fruit and veggies, and water routinely (every day)!

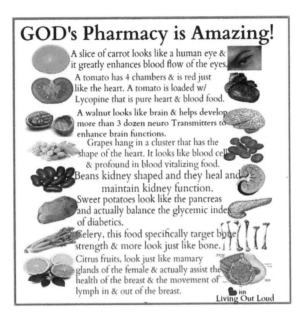

GOD's Pharmacy is Amazing!
A slice of carrot looks like a human eye & it greatly enhances blood flow of the eyes.
A tomato has 4 chambers & is red just like the heart. A tomato is loaded w/ Lycopine that is pure heart & blood food.
A walnut looks like brain & helps develop more than 3 dozen neuro Transmitters to enhance brain functions.
Grapes hang in a cluster that has the shape of the heart. It looks like blood cell & profound in blood vitalizing food.
Beans kidney shaped and they heal and maintain kidney function.
Sweet potatoes look like the pancreas and actually balance the glycemic index of diabetics.
Celery, this food specifically target bone strength & more look just like bone.
Citrus fruits, look just like mamary glands of the female & actually assist the health of the breast & the movement of lymph in & out of the breast.
isn
Living Out Loud

Constipation can be relieved in many ways. Most people know the routine, including fiber and produce. However, there is another way without consuming anything. When you are stretching especially in the heightened arched high back with your arms straight down knuckles on the floor, this stretches your abdomen and often even your colon. If you do this more than the routine thirty seconds, sometimes it will help. Some people even feel things moving inside. This stretch can give you the urge to eliminate sometimes only slightly, but helpful. Do extra sets.

Restless leg syndrome—many people have realized if they do not have any sugar after lunchtime, the restless leg syndrome goes away. This was the case for some of our children and me. Now eliminating all processed sugar has solved that problem completely.

Everything else you can imagine as illness or disease can benefit from following the plan in this book.

Research on the Body

Cells store sugar molecules as glycogen in animals and starch in plants; both plants and animals also use fats extensively as a food storage. These storage materials in turn serve as a major source of food for humans, along with the proteins that comprise the majority of the cells.

What should I eat for healthy cells?

- Antioxidants and aging—free radicals are molecules that can damage healthy cells.
- Berries—these are a great source of antioxidants and may help prevent cancer and some brain diseases.
- Olive oil—this tasty "good" fat may have anti-inflammatory and antioxidant properties.
- Fish.
- Beans.
- Vegetables.
- Nuts.
- Dairy.

Does your body make new cells from the food you eat? Yes. New cells are made to replace the old cells that become worn or damaged. Providing the raw materials for the creation of these new cells from the nutrients you get in your food is one way that nutrition plays an important role in sustaining your cellular and overall health.

When the stomach digests food, the carbohydrate (sugars and starches) in the food breaks down into another type of sugar called glucose. The stomach and small intestines absorb the glucose and then release it into the bloodstream.

Cells are generally soft, squishy, and easily damaged. However, many can repair themselves after being punctured, torn, or even ripped in half when damaged due to the normal wear-and-tear of normal physiology or as a result of injury or pathology, another case of your body healing itself.

When nutrient intake does not regularly meet the nutrient needs dictated by the cell activity, the metabolic processes slow down or even stop. In other words, nutrients give our bodies instructions about how to function. In this sense, food can be seen as a source of "information" for the body.

What's important to remember is that smoking and other harmful things going into your body produce substances called free radicals that attack healthy cells. When these healthy cells are weakened, they are more susceptible to cardiovascular disease and certain types of cancers.

Viruses are like hijackers. They invade living, normal cells and use those cells to multiply and produce other viruses like themselves. This can kill, damage, or change the cells and make you sick. Different viruses attack certain cells in your body such as your liver, respiratory system, or blood. This is why a healthy immune system is so important.

Foods that kill viruses:

- Elderberry
- Echinacea
- Garlic
- Green tea
- Licorice
- Olive leaf
- Pau D'Arco is a dietary supplement made from the inner bark of several species of Tabebuia trees that grow in Central and South America. I personally don't consume any supplements, except occasionally a whole food fruit or vegetable concentrated powder. A great one is Juice Plus. I also go for long periods of time with no supplements.

Bacteria and viruses thrive on sugar. It's their only source of energy. So consuming sweet snacks when you're sick can often make you feel worse. Sugar is bad for many reasons.

Top healthiest foods on earth:

- Spinach
- Black beans
- Walnuts
- Beets
- Avocado
- Raspberries
- Garlic

Six regenerative foods

1. Blueberries, raspberries, blackberries all help build up the powerful antioxidant superoxide dismutase (SOD). This is excellent for reducing oxidative stress, a key factor in liver support and the prevention of joint pain. Berries are also rich in flavonoids that reduce inflammation and repair cellular damage.
2. Broccoli is a cruciferous vegetable rich in sulforaphane, a chemical that increases enzymes in the liver, which work to neutralize the harmful toxins we breathe. All cruciferous vegetables are packed with a unique molecule called indole-3-carbinol that reduces inflammatory agents in the blood.
3. Ginger root is known for settling upset stomachs, but it also combats inflammation by inhibiting the effects of arachidonic acid, a necessary fat that triggers the inflammatory response.
4. Nuts and seeds—these healthy snacks have fats and protein to keep you full longer and satisfy cravings. Nuts are high in alpha-linolenic acid which is a type of anti-inflammatory omega-3 fat. Seeds contain plant sterols, known for their anti-inflammatory properties as well. I do recommend that you consume ground seeds, so there will be no problem in the colon.

5. Mushrooms like shiitake and maitake are high in polyphenols. These are nutrients known to help protect liver cells from damage by detoxifying them. Keeping the liver detoxified is critical in fighting inflammation because this is where we filter out toxins and break down our hormones.

6. Fatty fish and seafood—seafood contains eicosapentaenoic acid, a powerful anti-inflammatory type of omega-3 fatty acid. Studies show the oil in fish can act in an anti-inflammatory manner.

It's very important to incorporate these foods into your daily diet and to also "eat the rainbow" of organic fruit and vegetables in order to have complete nutrition and continual cell regeneration. Remember, if we think of food as medicine, then we open ourselves to a world of healing. A tooth is the *only* body part that cannot repair itself.

Some inquiring minds want to know the molecular structure, so for you the following is a snippet. Do atoms play a part? Cells are different from atoms and molecules. Atoms are not living things; they do not need food, water, and air, and they do not reproduce themselves. Cells are alive. Just as atoms have smaller parts called protons, neutrons, and electrons, cells have smaller parts. Cells are made up of atoms. However, the kinds of atoms that make up cells combine chemically to create particular molecules. The number of atoms per human cell is only a rough estimate because cells come in different sizes. Scientists estimate the average cell contains a hundred trillion atoms. The number of atoms per cell is about the same as the number of cells in the body.

Molecules are, by example, water, nitrogen, and even table salt. A molecule is the smallest particle in a chemical element or compound that has the chemical properties of that element or compound. Molecules are made up of atoms that are held together by chemical bonds. There are three food molecules: carbohydrates, proteins, and fats (all polymers). These molecules are major determinants of food texture and flavor; they are also essential for an array of physiological functions.

Although these are interesting facts, I have found nothing that tells me the plan in this book should not work for any person who is willing to dive fully into this concept. Every atom, molecule, and gravity is under God's control. Recognize that a sensation of pain is actually a signal for healing. A pain that signals serious long-term damage somewhere in your body is often the last symptom to appear. Meditation can cause a baseline for pain that is lower, but the diet seems to be primary. The diet helps you meditate correctly. Proficient meditators feel calm, centered, and at peace.

Following the instructions in the Bible, mainly following the fruit of the spirit, you can focus your energy on being happy. You are happy following a clean diet and core that gives you clarity. The core is always diet, sleep, and exercise.

Dedicate yourself to constant renewal daily. It does not hurt to try eliminating foods before spending time and money at the doctor's office. Optimal bodily health means that every cell in the body is performing and functioning properly and adequately. These functions are metabolism, repair, and work. We must feed our bodies at the cellular level. Basically, good health depends upon the integrity of metabolic function. It is important that one have, at all times, an adequate diet accompanied by good digestion and assimilation. Since your health is your most valuable asset, you cannot afford to avoid spending whatever time and energy is necessary to get to the truth concerning your underlying health. Then apply this truth to your daily life.

Wouldn't it be a wonderful feeling to awaken one bright morning and discover that you have no headache, no aches, and that you feel good all over and relaxed? What an experience to be filled with energy, good cheer, hopeful anticipation to greet the day and excited for the day.

Never look at someone who eats unhealthily but appears to be healthy as a guide. That person could be a ticking time bomb. People also have different metabolisms. These people may be able to assimilate unhealthy foods better than others. The unhealthy food usually takes its toll, if not now, later. Remember the people who live to be ninety and say they ate unhealthily, probably could have lived another ten or twenty healthy years and been happy if they had eaten healthy.

Good digestion begins in your mouth. This means that your mouth uses enzymes to do a certain job. We all need enzymes to do its job to be healthy. One entire book is written on this subject by Carlson Wade, *Helping your Health with Enzymes*. Although it goes in depth about enzymes, especially protein enzymes, it supports a clean healthy diet. Raw foods like fresh fruits and vegetables should be consumed daily. These will keep you young and healthy longer. *Fit for Life* book by Harvey and Marilyn Diamond was given to me by my brother Bill in the 80s. Some nuggets of this book are efficient absorption of food energy and efficient elimination of food bulk balance the body. The human body should last for 140 years. A more reasonable expectation may be 120 healthy years.

Use laughter, hope, faith, and love as primary help ingredients. Integrative medicine offers patients combinations of the traditional and the holistic (including diet, exercise, sunshine, rest, massage, and prayer). Integrative medicine regarding any disease is potentially reversible through the miraculous power of the body to heal itself.

Food fuel is most efficient in the form provided by nature, since our bodies are provided by nature. We know God made us. It is not only what you eat that makes a difference, but also of extreme importance is when you eat it and then in what combinations. I did not read many books for many hours on this particular subject because I listen to my body. If you pay attention to how your body reacts when you eat the good food and then in what combinations, you will have the answer quickly. The body is self-cleansing, self-healing, and self-maintaining, obviously if you give it the right nutrition.

Nine hundred miles south of Japan in Okinawa, there is the longest life expectancy on earth. Four hundred fifty of its citizens are age one hundred or older and healthy. They mainly have a plant food diet. They never overeat and put family first.

Age

In history, the Roman empire record shows adult life expectancy as twenty-eight years. Now it has risen to many years. When most people are thinking about living to seventy years of age, there's no reason another fifty years on average cannot be added to that life span. Twenty years ago, the oldest recorded life span was 121 years, an offshore Japanese islander. However, now many healthy Americans are living to that age.

This book was not written to help people live to a ripe old age or even lose weight, but they are good side effects. Mainly, the purpose is feeling good all the time and truly being healthy. Is it possible to be immune to illnesses? Many nutritional experts think yes. Remember nothing is impossible with God.

The hypothalamus is a tiny region of your brain no bigger than a fingertip, coordinates dozens of the body's automatic functions, earning it the nickname the brain brain. To help your automatic functions, your brain may be nourished with real whole food, and even your thinking. Think positive thoughts continuously.

All of these are natural and are in your body initially. I always said God made the perfect body, and we messed it up (changed it). We were made to be healthy and grow, not older deteriorating, but older in wisdom. There are dramatic instances where the man refused to believe in disease, and the body suddenly followed.

Of course, you are born with a specific body type. However, regardless of body type, consuming real whole food will help you. The plan in this book will greatly increase your odds in becoming healthy. Your perfect balance is a gift from God and is achievable.

Awareness has the capacity to heal. Of course, God is a miracle worker and can heal you, but why eat like a garbage truck when he has given you or at least offered you wisdom? Use your brain to make one decision to follow the plan in this book and receive the wisdom God wants in your life.

Fit for Life author says correct consumption means that fruit should never be eaten immediately following anything. It is essential when you eat fruit to eat it on an empty stomach. This is unquestionably the most important aspect of *Fit for Life*. I personally have not noticed any problem eating fruit anytime, but once again, people are different. See what works for you.

I can list all the fruits and vegetables that contain all the amino acids that produce what the body needs. However, you must select these based on your reaction after you eat them. They are carrots, bananas, brussels sprouts, cabbage, cauliflower, cucumbers, eggplant, kale, okra, peas, potatoes, summer squash, sweet potatoes, and tomatoes. Keep in mind that tomatoes, white potatoes, and even corn that can be included are foods most experts now say are not good for you. Once again, listen to your body.

Some experts say the only effect meat-eating has on health is that it deteriorates the body. Any day where fruits and vegetables are all you consume—and meat, grains, or dairy are not consumed at all—will be a high-energy maximum-weight-loss day. Many wonderful recipes are in the *Fit for Life* book.

Food that Heals

Since this book is not a compilation of other books but only has the nuggets from which you can choose, I am listing another book. *Foods that Heal* by Maureen Solomon has several interesting topics: twenty natural ways to lower cholesterol; five no-drug approaches to lowering high blood pressure; conquer your cravings for coffee, chocolate, tobacco, and alcohol, and lose weight the no-diet way. Beat arthritis, erase wrinkles, reverse aging effects with common foods.

People vary widely in how their bodies change over time. Researchers made the exciting discovery that the biological markers of aging can be retarded or even reversed through meditation. There are many good books on meditation by Dr. Robert Keith Wallace, PhD. People who meditate often report that they feel mentally and physically younger. Living in tune with nature means having healthy desires that match what you actually need.

Your instruction manual for life is the Bible. It is time tested, giving you pearls of wisdom. Love one another. Keep God's

Commandments. Seek and apply the fruit of the Spirit. Learn these nine fruits of the spirit, even though you have heard them many times. God wants you to be happy, and more importantly, have joy. Take time every day for relaxation. If you can, wake with the sun in the morning and watch the sunset in the evening.

Why does a person typically weigh the most at 7:00 p.m.? Probably because all has been consumed for the day and elimination occurs or should occur early in the morning. Scientists have now discovered these types of findings, and we can learn from them.

It is listening to your body and listening to the right signals. If you think your body is telling you that you really need ice cream, it is the wrong signal. Use the knowledge in this book and other books, if you prefer, to recognize the signals properly. Humans are made to sleep when it is dark. If your employment does not allow for this, make your environment the same as night when you sleep.

Elimination

During my police career, I witnessed many friends who told me they relied on coffee every morning so they could have a bowel movement. It certainly can work as a laxative. However, when cleaning your diet as recommended, you can eliminate caffeine. Therefore, you may want to drink some warm water each morning and allow approximately five minutes to see if you will have movement. Mine has been on track for so many years that it is routine after my fruit smoothie followed by one sixteen-ounce glass of room temperature water.

Now you are telling yourself this takes discipline. However, if approached with the right attitude, you will see it is exhilarating, exciting, and the benefits are boundless. Feeling good is not overrated. I tell you the truth, you need not feel bad.

The times to remove foods from your body are usually sugar two weeks, coffee three weeks, dairy three weeks, gluten three to four months, and alcohol eight days. Of course, the brain cells destroyed from the alcohol cannot be repaired.

Awareness

Meditation can have several descriptions. One is awareness. One such book about awareness is *Meta Human, Unleashing Your Infinite Potential* by Deepak Chopra, which is very interesting. The personal preference going beyond states this book is an invitation to find who you really are, beginning with two simple questions. In moments when you feel very happy, do you also watch yourself being happy? When you happen to get angry, is some part of you totally free of anger? If you answer yes to both questions you can stop reading (this section). You have arrived. Wow, I answered yes to both questions. It reinforced my plan in this book, starting with eating right.

Even in my law practice, my notice to client forms informing them of how the case will proceed, I give similar advice. "During your treatment, as well as other times, you should eat right (only good wholesome fruits, vegetables, etc., which will help your body heal), get enough sleep (preferably eight hours a night), exercise, including stretching (depending on your doctor's orders of course), and keep a healthy outlook (spiritual or focused optimistically) on life (in spite of the injury)."

This plan allows you to balance your whole system, including your physical body, mind, and soul. Soul is the master of all. It is the closest to God.

Most of your healing, and the best healing, occur when you sleep. If you follow the plan, you will achieve a lasting healing process. All of the children in my neighborhood, including me, received cuts, scrapes, and bruises periodically. My mom always said I was the fastest healer. Although my diet was not what it could be, I always slept a good night's sleep.

Don't gamble. Make conscious decisions to evolve over your remaining lifetime. Your good choices will radically upgrade your immunity to disease, slow down and reverse the aging process, and boost the healing response.

Instead of asking a friend for a referral, calling at least one doctor's office, waiting on the phone, waiting in the waiting room, raising your stress level about what will happen in the doctor's office, seeing the doctor only a few minutes when most, if not all, these days may seem disinterested, having your blood taken, and more blood taken than anyone could possibly need to check your levels, being given a prescription, which usually only treats the symptoms, having the insurance concern, paying your doctor bill or the full fee because it is not covered under your insurance, waiting for the receptionist to process your work, and needing to drive to get your prescription and, of course, waiting again there and paying more money, why not accept the role God gave you and take charge of your own life, saving all of this worry, time, and stress and be your own patient, loving, sympathetic, open-minded, knowledgeable healer? Don't question me thinking you can be knowledgeable about your healing. Everyone can get these answers quickly on the Internet. Often times, we are more fruitful in our application than the doctors.

Jesus told us in the Bible that we would actually do things mightier than he did when he was on earth. You know he healed the sick, blind, lame, and raised the dead. Did you ever think that he wants you to heal and save your own life physically as well as spiritually? The overall EAGLE plan will bring in balance the body, mind, and spirit. Remember, loving God is the priority. Find your spiritual path. This is exciting, fantastic stuff. Join the revolution.

If your illness has progressed, you will need to consult a physician. I hope you are able to find a qualified physician who uses a holistic plan in conjunction with other potential medical remedies. Don't dwell on the exceptions. Seize what you can do now. No amount of information can convince you that eating bad unhealthy food is good for you. Do you know this to be true? You simply need to take this knowledge, which is truthful, and apply it in your daily life. Do not panic. This is a simple one-step-at-a-time process.

There are many more holistic MDs today; however, I see patients still following the general MDs who routinely prescribe drugs and surgery. Some doctors may prescribe holistic measures, but the patients refuse to follow that route. I see now that it is actually the patients who require general MDs to prescribe drugs and surgery or simply choose not to follow the advice of holistic doctors.

Histology is the study of the microscopic structure of tissues. Holistic doctors seem to be more in line with how best to feed the tissues in our body. Look for a cure, not treatment for the symptoms. It is beyond me why a person chooses drugs and surgery without following alternative remedies first. The National Library of Medicine database has thousands of articles on alternative and complementary medicine with hundreds on herbal medicines alone.

Meditation, yoga, massage, exercise, and nutritional approaches are increasingly embraced as mainstream tools for healing. But once again, so many people are not willing to try these before drugs and surgery. Just like Joe Fox played by Tom Hanks in the movie *You've Got Mail,* opening the bookstore, he said, "We will get them in the end with 'our legally addictive stimulants,'" i.e., cappuccino.

Don't be ambivalent with your approach to seeking a healthier lifestyle. If needed, get paper and pen and write your plan. Review it each morning. Make a conscious decision to clean God's temple. Deepak Chopra says, "Self-knowledge will unfold for you every day." In time or perhaps at this very moment, you will see yourself living in the light. I absolutely see myself living in the light.

I have freedom from everything, except God. I choose to surrender to God because he absolutely wants what's best for us. My proposition is that if you truly love God, you will take care of his temple, your body, and prosper greatly. Do a daily devotional. Of all the apps you can have on your phone, install the Bible, with daily messages. My message today is "God is doing something incredible. And you can be a part of it." Do you not think that God can send me to help you?

It's estimated that the lack of physical activity in the US is costing $117,000,000,000 in annual health care. That's $117 billion! But taking a whack at that number is entirely possible given that only half of Americans are getting regular exercise. It's further estimated that one in fifteen cases of heart disease and one in twelve cases of diabetes could be prevented by some physical movement (Centers for Disease Control and Prevention). By just moving! You must keep moving daily!

It's a growth industry, and not necessarily in a good way. From 2012 to 2019, the rate of obesity in the US increased by eleven points and climbed to 30.8%. The state of Vermont ranks first as the healthiest with measurements below the national average, including both obesity and diabetes. Mississippi was the least healthy, with obesity rates nearing 40%. (America's health rankings, United Health Foundation).

The numbers on the horizon don't look a whole lot better. Projections by the Harvard T.H. Chan School of Public Health shows that obesity rate will grow to about *half of all Americans* by 2030. Some states might approach 60%, with even the lowest individual state rates nearing 40% by the next decade.

Need some good news? Rates for smoking mortality have driven downward since 1990, 43%. Public health initiatives have helped to decrease the rate of smoking, measuring 16.1% of American adults in 2019 (America's health rankings, Organization for Economic Cooperation and Development).

Americans spend about five hours a day in leisure activities, whether sports or socializing or just plain relaxing. But which activity ranks on top? The tube. Yes, watching TV sucks (3 hours a day from men and 2.61 hours from women, probably because men hog the remote). Reading consumes less than half an hour per day for each group (US Bureau of Labor Statistics). Other statistics show four hours of TV per day! This is why I know everybody can take time to be healthy.

I was already a nondrinker, consuming zero alcohol since I was young, exercising three times per week since my teens. This, of course, formed a habit toward living healthy. This is mentioned because so much of this book focuses on "as you get older," but young people should be starting now to clean your diet. You will thank me later.

In 1910, the availability of chicken and seafood to Americans was roughly the same, about ten pounds per person. That has since changed, with chicken soaring to number one. In 2017, 64.1 pounds of the white meat were available, outpacing beef by nearly 10 pounds. Fish and shellfish have increased to about 16.1 pounds per person (United States Department of Agriculture). Americans spend on average $9,450 per person annually on health care, but only $2,200 for food. Japanese spend $3,330 and $3,200 on health care and food respectively. What does that say about our priorities? My friend Randy McDaniel at lunch would ask health questions. Each time, I told him the answer was in my book. This book is written for Randy and all the other conscientious inquiring minds.

When considering quantum healing, at least four of the five senses are actually capable of experiencing the quantum domain directly, without the use of sophisticated scientific instruments. Einstein saw quantum theory as a means to describe nature on an atomic level, but he doubted that it upheld "a useful basis for the whole of physics." He thought that describing reality required firm predictions followed by direct observations. Einstein had his personal views about religion, and he believed in what he called "cosmic religion" where God's presence was evident in the order and rationality of nature and the universe in all its aspects and expressions. Chaos and randomness are, therefore, not part of nature (God does not play dice). Suffice it to say that we may be able to heal on a quantum level, but awareness seems to be the beginning to achieve healing of self.

Perfection

If you think you are perfect, with no problems whatsoever, still consuming a clean diet will ensure your future. There have been many people who thought they were healthy but were actually a ticking time bomb. Eating a clean healthy diet, it's never wrong.

Now that I have saved you from reading hundreds of books, take charge, love God by accepting his wisdom. Eat right, get enough sleep, exercise, and wash your hands. This is what God wants for your life. If you are healthy and alert, you can do more for him. That's what God wants, us being his eyes, ears, and hands. We are not each a Billy Graham, but we can do our part. Like the famous line in the *Star Wars* movie, stay on target!

In my almost forty years in the practice of law, I have routinely been the one to get up from the desk and move in the office. I will take files to the paralegal or secretary, walk to get files from them, always trying to stay in a relaxed and calm state. Movement is key.

Several courses called multitasking an ability. However, I think multitasking divides your attention, and it is difficult to give your full ability to any one task. Don't multitask. The more you are able to work in a quiet environment free of interruptions, better the work product.

Every thirty to sixty minutes, it is good to get up from your desk and walk. Annette Forlines in our office would routinely remind everyone to get up and stretch. This should allow some inter-action with other employees and the opportunity to recharge. This also stretches your muscles, which should be occurring continuously throughout your waking hours.

It is acceptable for you to be in love with your body. God made it. He made it in his image, and his desire is for you to treat it like his temple. I love God, and I love what he makes. When we love and feel that people love us, it is power. This power of love increases our self-esteem. Self-esteem leads us to take better care of ourselves. Ultimately, love creates a constant state of healing. I have always loved myself. Maybe that started when I was in the orphanage at such a young age (starting at age one and a half). Maybe it was a survival instinct created in the project in Atlanta to survive. Find your desire to achieve.

Following the plan in this book, what do you have to lose? You might think about some of the food you lose, but did you think you might lose the pain and potential surgeries and drugs? If you love others, and people love you, your healing self has a giant start.

Researchers have proven that people who argue have a lower immune system. If there is ever an argument, and we are human so that certainly can happen, close the door (figuratively) as fast as possible. When removing yourself from any argument, tell yourself, "I will not let that person rob my joy." Tell yourself even though you may be mad, that you are not going to let that bother you any longer. Don't have a war with yourself; but keep telling yourself to be calm, relaxed, and go to a quiet place where you can restore self.

God loves everything about you, he loves you. My friend Jerry Baker says, "God is big enough to hear anything you want to tell him." Don't ever run from God. Go to him as often as needed and give him any burden. I always say give God your prayer request without claw marks. That's what God tells us in his Word. Believe it and enjoy the reward.

The ultimate goal is not to do everything on your list but to do what you do in an efficient manner while creating happiness or joy. Psychologists learned that happy people have a strategy. That must be why each morning, when I wake, I decide, regardless of circumstances, it will be a good day, I will feel good, and I will be happy. I also ask God to help me look for those opportunities to help other people. This gives you the right perspective. It is all right to smile constantly and let people know that you are happy. You can still be concerned about the sick, shut-in, and needy; but do that in a positive happy way.

When you are fulfilling Scripture, you should be happy. Self-awareness can be a major component of a lifestyle that is healing itself. Upon completing this regimen, you will have no conflicts, no conflicts with yourself or with other people. Awareness or the wholeness of pure consciousness will give you clarity to make priorities. You will know this has occurred when you realize God must be first. Although there are many health books, this book connects health directly to God. Unfold the practical approach to getting healthy and how God intends for you to be healthy.

Doctors are not responsible for your health. Certainly, the pharmaceutical companies are not responsible for your health. The pharmacy gives you something that almost always only treats the symptoms. Now more than ever, the side effects can be worse than the reason you are taking the prescription. You, and you alone, are responsible for your health. The good news is that the secrets of self-healing are actually very simple. It is urgent and mandatory for you to follow these simple guidelines to obtain optimum health. Destroy what will destroy you (before it acts first). If not this, what? If not now, when? If not you, who?

Miracles happen! When you have health, you have hope. Albert Einstein once said, "There are two ways to live your life. One is as though nothing is a miracle. The other is as though everything is a miracle." I pray this book is a miracle.

Knowledge brings choices, and choices bring opportunities. You have the power, authority, and ability to transform your health for the better. Genes will imprint you from birth, and even behavior and environment will imprint you before you have the ability to successfully choose. However, we can change this imprint by choosing beliefs, behaviors, and interpretations we actually desire.

As you age, your body is being transformed. Whether you like it or not, you will be transformed by your cravings or your intent. Your intent to be healthy and happy can allow your brain to control your body. This knowledge is useless unless you act upon it. Like that song by Chicago *Feeling Stronger Every Day*, you will. Join the revolution. It is better if you have a partner or friend who can help keep you accountable while you change your lifestyle. However, I have been alone in this journey all my life and proven it can be done individually.

Would you like to eat anything you want and still be healthy? Absolutely. Following the program outlined in this book allows you to do that. In the process, it changes your thinking. I eat anything and everything I want every day. The difference is I do not want garbage. I call fried foods and other very unhealthy foods garbage. They are. I do not know anyone happier than I am. That is because once you clean your diet, you will only want and desire the healthy foods. You will have peace that comes from God, which does pass all understanding.

Scriptures and Inspiration

For God so loved the world that he gave his one and only son, that whoever believes in him shall not perish but have eternal life. (John 3:16, New International Version)

Jesus answered, "I am the way and the truth and the life. No one comes to the Father except through me" [in response to Thomas asking how to know the way]. (John 14:6).

Therefore, I urge you brothers, in view of God's mercy, to offer your bodies as living sacrifices, holy and pleasing to God, this is your spiritual act of worship. Do not conform any longer to this world, but be transformed by the renewing of your mind. Then you will be able to test and approve what God's will is, his good, pleasing and perfect will. [This means to surrender to God.] (Romans 12:1–2)

[Have I not commanded you?] Be strong and courageous. Do not be terrified; do not be discouraged, for the Lord your God will be with you wherever you go. (Joshua 1:9)

When I am filled with cares, your comfort brings me joy. (Psalm 94:19)

Delight yourself in the Lord and he will give you the desires of your heart. (Psalm 37:4)

May the God of hope fill you with all joy and peace as you trust in him, so that you may overflow with hope by the power of the Holy spirit. (Romans 14:13)

PERSONAL NOTE

Although I am one of eleven, it is not as it sounds. My parents divorced before I was born. Each remarried and had six children. I am the only common link.

I never used a sick day at work in my life. I was sick during my youth like everybody else but never sick enough to miss work. There were days when I used a vacation day to rest or recuperate. I was raised in the days when you did not want to miss work. If you did miss, you did not get paid, end of story.

Later, when sick days were offered, the employer also provided if you did not use a sick day, you would be paid a portion of the sick time not used and the same time was saved for a later date. Upon retiring from the Atlanta Police Department, I had all my sick days and retired early. Maybe we need an incentive to be healthy. I think feeling good every day is enough incentive.

My dad would often say there's only one difference in life, knowing and not knowing. You now know how to do it. You are in a different position. Choose wisely.

CONCLUSION

Could some people be born with the ability to live healthy? Perhaps. However, if you think you were not born with the ability to be healthy, you can still be healthy. By telling yourself you can be healthy and exercising that attitude, you can build on that to become resilient. The way to being healthy can be learned. This book offers you that chance.

There is a song at church, "I'm free indeed, in Christ I'm free indeed, no chains are holding me, it's who I choose to be." There is a lot of truth in that. If you choose to be free and believe it, you are on the right track. The next stanza repeats and then ends with, "It's who I'm meant to be." True again. God made you to be free. Claim it! The willpower you can acquire not only gives you the power and ease of eating healthy but will give you willpower for all aspects of life.

Making God choices is actually easy. He created you in his image. He created you to choose him. We find many other reasons not to do so, but we have an innate desire to love and serve God. It is important for you to understand and apply this principle.

So what does it mean to balance genetics, environment, your mental health, physical, including EAGLE, and decide where to start? It absolutely can start with what goes in your mouth. Follow the total plan in this book if you want to truly be healthy. Then you will achieve the true perfect balance that will make you healthy and happy.

Be an EAGLE!
Eat right.
Always get enough sleep.

Get to exercising.
Love cleanliness.
Especially love God.

I pray that each reader will follow the easy steps in this book and be healthy and happy. God bless you always.

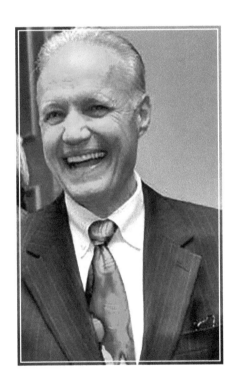

ACKNOWLEDGMENTS

I am thankful to all who supported me:

To God for giving the fruit of the Spirit and Jesus who is truth, for allowing me to be a part of the big picture, salvation.

My wife, Pam Moore, who has been the most caring person and will always be the love of my life. Although she questions much of my endeavors, she supports my decisions. Thank you for being my partner.

Family, especially our children. Mine: Reba, Dave (Walter David), Fawn, and Candice. Pam's: Mandi, Lauren, and Davie (David Earl). Their attributes are numerous, but primarily Reba for her gift of compassion, Dave for laughter, Fawn for courage, Candice for innocence, Mandi for adventure, Lauren for authenticity, and Davie for persistence. My mom for faith and dad for strength and service.

My best health mentor on this journey for many years is Dr. Rachel Smartt, ND, who penned the foreword in this book. She has inspired me and countless others to strive to be the best we can be by eating healthy. She constantly lives her passion, and it shows in how she helps others. Rachel rises above all others with a lifestyle change that is the epitome of the pursuit of happy and healthy.

Legal mentors William J. (Bill) McKenney, Tim Hall, Adam Collins, Chris Edwards, Pete Law, Gibson Vance, Rob Register, Adam Malone, Tommy Malone, Mark Skibiel, Durance Lowendick, Don Keenan, Jack Hinton, and Scott Walters.

My law partners Larry Melnick, Michael Brennan, Ken Green, Jim Brown, Sheila Huddleston, Daniel Kalamaro, David Ballard,

Michael Burnett, James Clifton, Dan Gibbs, Jennifer Roberts, Stephen Ott, Richard Elliott, and Cliff Milam have made life in the practice fun, which has reduced stress (to about zero).

Spiritual hero Kenneth Pope (and the entire Pope family) drove a bus from the other side of Atlanta for years to the inner-city project to take us heathen children to church. That is when I accepted Christ at age twelve, which of course, changed my life for the better forever.

Accountability partner John Whitworth has been meeting with me for a quarter of a century and investing in my spiritual growth, holding me accountable to God. John Martin Maund for being accountable with me and encouraging me continuously.

Quinton King is a lawyer and Christian, who inspired me to be the best Christian lawyer possible. He is the hero who always sets the example of Christ serving others.

Spiritual mentors Jerry Baker, Libby Baker, Barry Babb, Tina Plunkett, Bob and Linda Dukes, Lee Haney, Rebecca Paugh, Charles Warr, and many Sunday school teachers have poured into me spiritually.

Spiritual leaders John Avant, Rhys Stenner, Tim Woodruff, Hugh Kirby, John Conrad, Dan Cathy, David Anders, Talmadge French, Ryan French, Nathan French, Al Mead, Woody Johnson, Rich Terry, Mike Yonkers, Vandy Pope, Jerry Young, Jim Hardee, Perry Stone, Lee Brewer, Franklin Graham, Jentzen Franklin, Robby Zacharias, David Jerimiah, Billy Graham, Ron Jansen, Charles Stanley, Andy Stanley, Joel Osteen, Joyce Meyers, Beth Moore, Irvin Baxter, Kenneth Morgan, Tom Burdett, and John Hagee.

To my professional and civic organizations, especially Peachtree City Rotary, Fayette and Atlanta Bar Associations, State Bar of Georgia, and the Fayette Chamber of Commerce.

Publisher: Christian Faith Publishing.

Editor: a special thank-you to Dr. David Anders for assisting with some of the initial editing.

Illustrations assistance by Candice Moore.

ENDORSEMENTS

Written by a layman, *Perfect Balance* proves that one need not be a reverend or a doctor to gain valuable insights for an intentionally successful, spiritually rewarding, and healthy life. David Moore will challenge some of your beliefs and strengthen others, which is always a good formula for the never-ending pursuit of self-improvement. Condensed from his reading of hundreds of health books and religious interpretive books, David Moore dispenses bite-sized "gold nuggets." His challenge to the reader is, "We are different, so see what works best for you." As you read, some nuggets you'll savor, and others may seem a bitter pill to swallow. But each is served up with the hope of having you realize a conscious choice is made every day to determine whether you will be a turkey or an EAGLE. As one of those "general MDs" (i.e., not primarily holistic) with whom he sometimes finds disfavor, you can decide for yourself where he and I agree and where we might differ. (Spoiler alert, he best sums it up toward the end: "Now that I have saved you from reading hundreds of books, take charge, love God by accepting His wisdom, eat right, get enough sleep, exercise, and wash your hands." But he has so much more to say, so start reading now!)

David L. Anders, MD, FACP
Board Certified by the American Board of Internal Medicine:
Internal Medicine, Geriatrics, and
Hospice and Palliative Medicine

David Moore offers a balanced and biblical way of living a life of good health and wisdom. *Perfect Balance* is filled with practical advice gleaned from personal experience and offered in simple, proverbial statements that capture the essence of wholeness and wellbeing. I heartily recommend this book as an inspiration for establishing good habits for a healthy body and flourishing soul. It will be an often quoted and referenced repository that supports a life well lived.

Robert D. (Bob) Dukes,
President and executive director
Worldwide Discipleship Association

Perfect Balance is a compendium of knowledge acquired from medical, psychological, and theological wisdom, as well as Attorney David Moore's considerable observations about life. He presents his insights in easily digestible nuggets like the Proverbs or *Poor Richard's Almanack*. This volume is a practical guide not just to living but to living well. It can be read by complete chapters or by paging through and honing in upon quick, easy-to-follow suggestions. By modifying a few behaviors and attitudes a month, in no time, you can be soaring like an EAGLE.

David Aycock, PhD
Licensed psychologist
A New Start Counseling Center, Inc.

David Moore and *Perfect Balance*. I have known David for years; and his life is certainly one of faith, service, and healthy energy. He gives us insights that are true in his life, not dry theories but practical principles and advice. David practices what he preaches. You may not agree with everything here, but you will definitely receive an excellent pathway for a life of faith, health, and wellbeing. *Perfect Balance* is a resource that you will want to keep close by for regular coaching to be a good steward of the life God has given you.

Tim Woodruff, EdD
Executive pastor, Ministry Development
New Hope Baptist Church

Perfect Balance contains the nuggets of wisdom from hundreds of health books and religious interpretive books, as well as personal life experiences. It also removes the superfluous material that might hinder you getting a grasp of what's important. I am impressed with the wisdom, dedication, and encouragement contained in this book. I implore you to read this book and implement David's suggestions. The payoffs will be well worth the price of sacrifice. When you have health, anything is possible; and without it, nothing else really matters.

Dr. Rachel Smartt, ND, smartttransformations.com
Author, speaker, plant-base coach, nutritional counselor
Peachtree City, Georgia

I have the honor and privilege of knowing David Moore for over twenty years. David and his wife Pam have been deeply involved in serving our church in Fayetteville, Georgia, and my wife and I love them dearly. I have read a lot of books on health and fitness through the years. I was blessed to be involved in competitive sports for over fifty years. I do not think I have ever seen a more practical and comprehensive book on health and fitness. David gives his readers a well-rounded look at the physical, mental, emotional, and spiritual insights of how to live life and live it abundantly. I highly recommend *Perfect Balance.*

Hugh Kirby,
Intergenerational minister
New Hope Baptist Church

ABOUT THE AUTHOR

From rags to riches, David, who was one of eleven, was raised in poverty in the inner-city projects in Atlanta. He rose to become the most decorated police officer in the Atlanta Police Department, receiving Officer of the Year, Employee of the Year (for all four departments), and the Mayoral Award. After retiring from law enforcement, he became a successful lawyer in Atlanta and has managed his own firm, now twelve lawyers, for over a quarter of a century. David credits this to God. He says God allowed him to choose, and he has persevered regardless of circumstances.

CPSIA information can be obtained
at www.ICGtesting.com
Printed in the USA
LVHW012300190122
708244LV00006B/23